SLAY THE CLAIMS DENIAL DRAGON

HOW TO REVERSE AS MANY DENIED INSURANCE CLAIMS AS WIZARDLY POSSIBLE

By

Rebecca Hollinger & Don Kermath

The Revenue Recovery Wizards

D1712947

1

Copyright Warning and Disclaimer

TABLE OF CONTENTS

IMPORTANT! READ THIS FIRST

Dear Friend,

Embarking on the journey through this book "Slay the Claims Denial Dragon: How to Reverse as Many Denied Insurance Claims as Wizardly Possible" will be the catalyst for a transformation in your revenue recovery strategy.

Much like our previous book, "15 Money-Murdering Mistakes No Medical Billing Company Would Dare to Tell You: Plus the Mistake That Will Kill Your Practice," this edition is tailored to address a critical challenge faced by healthcare providers — the bane of denied insurance claims.

We've witnessed denied claims drain millions from healthcare coffers, and conversely, our guidance has propelled our clients to earn millions in revenue.

Reversing a denied claim is ten times more challenging than processing it accurately the first time. This realization led us to craft a dedicated guide for unraveling the intricacies of denied claims.

"Slay the Claims Denial Dragon" is a wizardly solution applicable to healthcare providers of all sizes and specialties. We firmly believe that every provider deserves a strategy that safeguards revenue and minimizes the impact of denied claims.

Here are four core reasons why our Denial Reversal Method is a force to be reckoned with:

1. **Comprehensive Insight**: Gain a profound understanding of common pitfalls in reversing denied claims, empowering you to identify and rectify errors proactively.

2. **Practical Solutions**: Discover actionable steps for immediate implementation, fortifying your billing accuracy and averting potential errors.

3. **Expert Guidance**: Benefit from the expertise of the Revenue Recovery Wizards, who bring deep insights into the medical billing landscape, providing guidance that is both practical and invaluable.

4. **Proven Results**: Our Denial Reversal Method is not theoretical; it's been put to the test and has yielded significant results for healthcare providers, ensuring a path to revenue maximization.

As you read this book you are going to realize the information is worth hundreds of thousands if not millions of dollars. You're going to wonder why we are sharing our Denial Reversal Method for such a low price.

You know, our main goal is to tackle the ongoing opioid crisis that's been causing so many problems in our society. What we're really focused on is helping the amazing people who work in behavioral health and substance use centers. We want to support them in providing as much treatment as they can.

To do that, these centers need to get as much money as possible from insurance companies, Medicaid, and Medicare. The more money they get from these sources, the less they have to ask their patients to pay. And that's important because these patients are going through a really tough time, trying to overcome addiction.

Our time is scarce. We can only help dozens of providers every year serving thousands of patients. But with a book, we can share our expertise with thousands of providers serving hundreds of thousands of patients.

This is our small way of addressing the crippling ongoing opioid crisis.

No matter what kind of healthcare you provide and no matter where you are on your journey, we hope this book turns out to be magically helpful.

Thank you for giving us the opportunity to help you.

Magically Yours,

Rebecca and Don, The Revenue Recovery Wizards

P.S. The real magic happens when you implement the action items promptly as you progress through each chapter.

"And so, castles made of sand slips into the sea, eventually." — *Jimi Hendrix*

INTRODUCTION TO OLD ACCOUNTS RECEIVABLE RECOVERY

Welcome to the ultimate guide to old accounts receivable recovery! In this comprehensive guide, we'll walk you through the step-by-step process of recovering old accounts receivable and reclaiming the revenue you deserve.

Whether you're a healthcare provider, medical practice manager, or billing professional, this guide is packed with actionable strategies and expert insights to help you navigate the intricate world of accounts receivable and achieve financial success.

UNDERSTANDING THE IMPORTANCE OF OLD AR RECOVERY

In the labyrinthine realm of medical billing, a distinctive journey awaits—one that ventures into the heart of financial recovery and practices vitality. Embarking upon this expedition unveils the profound significance of Old Accounts Receivable (AR) Recovery—a quest laden with promises of rediscovered revenue and strengthened financial fortitude.

THE IMPACT OF UNRECOVERED REVENUE ON YOUR PRACTICE

Amidst the cascading currents of your practice's operations, the specter of unrecovered revenue lurks ominously. It is a force that casts a shadow upon your financial landscape, limiting your potential and constraining your ability to thrive. Let us illuminate the consequences of this elusive revenant, drawing the curtain back to reveal the stark truths.

Stifled Growth and Innovation

Unrecovered revenue acts as a formidable barrier, curtailing your practice's ability to innovate, expand services, and embrace transformative technologies. It confines your growth within a stifling cocoon, impeding your evolution into a dynamic healthcare provider.

Eroded Profit Margins

The specter of unrecovered revenue siphons away the hard-earned fruits of your labor. As resources are squandered in the mist of neglect, profit margins erode, weakening your practice's financial foundation.

Compromised Patient Care

The unrecovered revenue phantom sows seeds of

uncertainty in the fertile ground of patient care. Diminished resources translate to compromised services, leaving patients in the shadows of unfulfilled potential.

Operational Strain

The burden of unrecovered revenue places undue strain upon your administrative machinery. Resources that could be harnessed to streamline operations are instead channeled toward the quagmire of overlooked financial opportunities.

Missed Investment Opportunities

Every uncollected dollar is a lost opportunity—a missed chance to invest in advanced medical equipment, staff development, or enhanced patient experiences. The specter of unrecovered revenue stands as a sentinel, guarding the gateway to these transformative possibilities.

Blighted Provider-Patient Relationships

The ripple effect of unrecovered revenue extends beyond finances, infiltrating the realm of provider-patient relationships. As the fabric of trust frays, patient loyalty wanes, and the symbiotic bond between healer and healed is tarnished.

With these revelations, the significance of Old AR Recovery emerges as a beacon of hope—a path to rekindling the flames of potential, reclaiming lost resources, and nurturing the very essence of your practice's prosperity.

In the chapters that follow, we shall unveil the arcane wisdom of Old AR Recovery, each chapter a portal into the mystical techniques and profound strategies wielded by the Revenue Recovery Wizards. Brace yourself, for this journey shall illuminate the shadows, dissolve the revenant of unrecovered revenue, and guide you toward the radiant shores of financial rejuvenation.

ACTION ITEMS

1. **Self-Assessment of Revenue Health:** Take a moment to evaluate the overall financial health of your practice. Look at the percentage of old accounts receivable and identify any patterns of unpaid claims or denied reimbursements.

2. **Identify Revenue Goals:** Define clear financial goals for recovering old accounts receivable. Determine the percentage of revenue you aim to recover from these accounts and set a timeframe for achieving these goals.

3. **Understanding Denial Impact:** Examine the impact of denied claims and unpaid accounts on your practice's financial stability. Calculate the potential revenue loss over time due to these challenges.

4. **Assess Current Recovery Efforts:** Evaluate your existing strategies for old AR recovery, if any. Identify what's working well and what areas need improvement.

5. **Educate Your Team:** Share the importance of old AR recovery with your billing and administrative staff. Discuss how effective recovery can positively impact the practice's financial future.

6. **Review Current Processes:** Analyze your current billing and reimbursement processes to identify bottlenecks or potential causes of denied claims. Look for areas that can be streamlined and

improved.

7. **Set Priorities:** Determine which unpaid claims or denied reimbursements require immediate attention. Prioritize based on factors such as dollar value, claim age, and potential for successful recovery.

8. **Commit to Improvement:** Embrace a proactive attitude toward old AR recovery. Make a commitment to implementing the strategies outlined in this guide and working toward a healthier revenue cycle.

9. **Gather Data:** Start collecting data on common denial reasons, recurring issues, and patterns in old accounts receivable. This information will be invaluable as you refine your recovery strategies.

10. **Stay Open-Minded:** Approach the upcoming chapters with an open mind, ready to learn new techniques and strategies for enhancing your practice's financial well-being.

11. **Engage with the Guide:** Dedicate time to thoroughly read and understand each chapter of the guide. Take notes on key concepts, potential solutions, and ideas that resonate with your practice's needs.

12. **Actionable Takeaways:** As you progress through each chapter, identify actionable takeaways that can be immediately implemented in your practice. Start envisioning how these changes will positively impact your revenue recovery efforts.

13. **Seek Internal Support:** Rally support from key stakeholders within your practice, including administrators, billing staff, and providers. Collaboration and commitment are crucial for successful old AR recovery.

14. **Embrace a Positive Mindset:** Approach the challenge of old AR recovery with a positive mindset. Understand that this journey will lead to increased financial stability and improved patient care.

15. **Prepare for Change:** Embrace the mindset that improvement requires change. Be open to adopting new processes and strategies to better your practice's financial health.

16. **Take the First Step:** Prepare yourself mentally and emotionally to embark on this journey of old AR recovery. The path may have obstacles, but with determination, you can overcome them and pave the way to financial success.

Remember, old accounts receivable recovery is a dynamic process that demands ongoing attention and adaptation. The action items outlined here will set you on the path to a successful recovery journey, ultimately enhancing your practice's financial well-being.

COMMON CHALLENGES IN OLD AR RECOVERY

UNRAVELING THE ENIGMA OF UNPAID CLAIMS

Amid the intricate tapestry of medical billing, a symphony of challenges weaves a melody of complexity, and none is more haunting than the echoes of unpaid claims.

As we embark on this expedition through the labyrinthine landscape of Old Accounts Receivable (AR) Recovery, let us cast a light upon the common challenges that often entwine and obscure the path to financial restoration.

IDENTIFYING THE ROOT CAUSES OF UNPAID CLAIMS

Behold the first veil concealing the secrets of unrecovered revenue—the enigmatic root causes of unpaid claims. These elusive culprits, concealed within the folds of labyrinthine transactions, hold the key to unlocking the doors of financial reclamation.

Coding Conundrums

As if deciphering an ancient script, the correct translation of medical services into precise codes is paramount. Yet, this task is fraught with perils—misinterpretations, inaccuracies, and oversights lurk in the shadows, transforming claims into denials. We shall delve deep into the mystic arts of accurate coding to unveil the remedy for these arcane afflictions.

Documentation Dilemmas

The chronicler's quill must paint a vivid portrait of each patient encounter—a tale of medical necessity and care. Yet, incomplete or cryptic documentation obscures this narrative, leaving claims vulnerable to the dark specter of denial. Through our journey, the incantations of comprehensive documentation shall be revealed, banishing the shadows of insufficient record-keeping.

Compliance Curses

The realm of medical billing is governed by an intricate web of regulations and guidelines, a realm where a single misstep can invoke the ire of compliance denials. The path to restoration lies in mastering these arcane rules, ensuring that your practice navigates the labyrinth with utmost precision.

ADDRESSING DENIAL PATTERNS AND TRENDS

Beyond the labyrinthine veil of root causes, a tapestry of denial patterns and trends emerges—each thread representing a unique challenge to your practice's revenue flow. As we unravel these intricate patterns, the path to successful Old AR Recovery becomes clearer, and the arcane dance of claim resolution is revealed.

The Denial Alchemy

Denials manifest as the alchemical result of numerous ingredients—coding discrepancies, documentation gaps, and administrative oversights. We shall decode these formulas, transforming denials into actionable insights for financial rejuvenation.

Trend Analysis Sorcery

Within the vast expanse of denied claims lies a hidden treasure—patterns and trends that, when deciphered, hold the keys to prevention. Our wizardry will equip you to unveil these trends, empowering your practice to proactively shield itself from recurring denials.

The Elixir of Resolution

Denials need not be the final verdict—resolution is the elixir that transforms them into successful claims. Our journey will illuminate the mystical rituals of appeals, guiding you in your quest to overturn denials and reclaim rightful revenue.

Prepare yourself, intrepid traveler, for the path ahead is fraught with challenges and mysteries. Yet, fear not, for each challenge presents an opportunity to hone your skills, wield newfound wisdom, and navigate the labyrinth of Old AR Recovery with the finesse of a true Revenue Recovery Wizard.

ACTION ITEMS

1. **Analyze Denial Trends:** Review your historical denied claims to identify recurring denial patterns. Categorize denials based on common reasons such as coding errors, missing documentation, or incorrect patient details.

2. **Data-Driven Insights:** Utilize data analytics tools to gain insights into your practice's denial rates, aging AR accounts, and reimbursement trends. This information will help you pinpoint the areas needing improvement.

3. **Evaluate Workflow Processes:** Examine your existing billing and claims submission workflow. Identify any bottlenecks or inefficiencies that might contribute to claim denials and unpaid accounts.

4. **Conduct Root Cause Analysis:** For a representative sample of denied claims, perform a thorough root cause analysis to understand the underlying issues. This will guide your efforts to develop targeted solutions.

5. **Educate Your Team:** Share the identified denial patterns and common challenges with your billing and administrative team. This awareness can lead to more proactive claim handling and prevention of future issues.

6. **Implement Training Programs:** Offer training sessions for your billing staff on specific denial prevention and recovery strategies. Keep them

informed about industry updates and best practices.

7. **Adopt Denial Tracking Tools:** Invest in denial tracking software or tools that can help you monitor and manage the status of denied claims. Use these tools to track progress and measure improvements.

8. **Define Accountability:** Assign responsibility for handling specific denial categories or stages of recovery. Clearly define roles and expectations within your team to ensure consistent follow-up.

9. **Develop Denial Prevention Protocols:** Create detailed protocols for your billing team to follow when submitting claims. These protocols should address common denial triggers and emphasize accurate data entry and documentation.

10. **Regular Review Meetings:** Schedule regular meetings to review denied claims and old AR accounts with your team. Collaboratively brainstorm solutions and share insights from each team member's experiences.

11. **Engage with Payers:** Open lines of communication with insurance companies to understand their specific denial reasons and requirements. Seek clarification on complex cases and work toward mutual understanding.

12. **Set Benchmark Metrics:** Define key performance indicators (KPIs) related to denial rates, recovery percentages, and account aging. Regularly monitor these metrics and use them to track progress.

13. **Tailor Solutions to Patterns:** Develop customized solutions for addressing specific denial patterns. These could include process

improvements, enhanced documentation, or payer-specific strategies.

14. **Invest in Technology:** Explore technological solutions like AI-powered claims scrubbing tools or electronic claim submission platforms that can reduce the likelihood of errors and denials.

15. **Regularly Update Policies:** Keep your billing policies and procedures up to date with the latest industry regulations and payer requirements. This proactive approach can prevent future challenges.

16. **Collaborate with Providers:** Foster collaboration between billing and healthcare providers to ensure accurate documentation and coding, reducing the risk of denial due to incomplete or incorrect information.

17. **Share Best Practices:** Encourage knowledge sharing among your billing team members. Regularly discuss best practices and success stories to inspire continuous improvement.

18. **Feedback Loop Implementation:** Establish a feedback loop where your billing team can report issues or potential challenges that lead to denials. Use this information to drive process improvements.

19. **Celebrate Small Wins:** Recognize and celebrate instances of successful denial recovery or prevention. This positive reinforcement can motivate your team to stay committed to improving the process.

20. **Continuous Improvement Culture:** Foster a culture of continuous improvement by encouraging your team to seek innovative solutions and embrace change. Regularly revisit and refine your strategies based on outcomes.

Remember, tackling the common challenges in old AR recovery requires a multi-faceted approach. By implementing these action items, you can lay a solid foundation for addressing denials and improving the recovery process in your practice.

BUILDING YOUR RECOVERY STRATEGY

FORGING YOUR PATH TO FINANCIAL RESTORATION

In the realm of Old Accounts Receivable (AR) Recovery, every step taken is a deliberate stride toward the reclamation of untapped revenue. As we embark on this journey, let us wield the wisdom of the Revenue Recovery Wizards to craft a formidable strategy—a roadmap that navigates the twists and turns of the recovery landscape.

SETTING CLEAR GOALS AND OBJECTIVES

Behold, the cornerstone of your expedition—the beacon that guides your every move. Setting clear goals and objectives is the first spell to cast, imbuing your endeavor with purpose and direction.

The Alchemical Transformation

Envision the metamorphosis you seek—whether it be a specific monetary goal, a reduction in aged AR, or the enhancement of your revenue cycle. Define the essence of your pursuit and let it crystallize into a tangible goal that shall serve as your North Star.

The Elixir of Clarity

The wizard's path is illuminated by clarity. Outline your objectives with precision, delineating the milestones that mark your progress. Each step forward shall bring you closer to the ultimate enchantment—financial restoration.

PRIORITIZING ACCOUNTS FOR RECOVERY

Amidst the myriad threads of aged AR lies a tapestry woven with opportunity. To unravel it effectively, one must wield the wand of discernment and prioritize accounts with sagacious intent.

The Enchanted Sorting Hat

Let the Sorting Hat of Prioritization guide your hand. Categorize accounts based on factors such as dollar value, payer type, or aging period. Unveil the accounts that harbor the greatest potential for swift recovery and weave your spells accordingly.

The Whispering Wind of Analysis

Listen closely to the whispering wind of data analysis. Study denial patterns, historical performance, and potential roadblocks. These insights shall reveal the accounts worthy of immediate attention and ensure that your efforts yield maximum returns.

CREATING A STRUCTURED RECOVERY PLAN

In the arcane dance of Old AR Recovery, structure is your ally—a magical framework that channels your energies and harnesses your efforts. Craft your recovery plan with meticulous care, for it shall serve as the map that guides you through the labyrinth of reclamation.

The Scroll of Action

Unfurl the Scroll of Action—a comprehensive plan that outlines each step of your recovery journey. Detail the actions required, assign responsibilities and set deadlines. Let the scroll be your constant companion, ensuring that no opportunity is overlooked.

The Weaving of Timelines

Weave timelines into the fabric of your plan, for time is the currency of recovery. Determine when each action shall unfold and create a cadence that keeps momentum alive. Your structured approach shall transform ambition into achievement.

The Resonance of Collaboration

Call upon the resonance of collaboration to unite your team under a common purpose. Forge alliances with coders, billers, and administrators, pooling your collective expertise to overcome challenges and amplify success.

As you forge your path to financial restoration, remember that every incantation cast, every objective set, and every step taken is a testament to your dedication as a true Revenue Recovery Wizard. Embrace the power of clear goals, the wisdom of prioritization, and the magic of structure, for they shall propel you toward the reclamation of revenue long entwined in the labyrinthine threads of Old AR.

ACTION ITEMS

1. **Define Clear Recovery Goals:** Identify specific goals for your recovery efforts, such as reducing AR aging or increasing recovery percentages. Ensure these goals are measurable and aligned with your practice's financial objectives.

2. **Analyze Historical Data:** Review historical data on old AR accounts, denial rates, and recovery trends. This analysis will help you prioritize accounts and understand where recovery efforts are needed most.

3. **Segment Your Accounts:** Categorize old AR accounts based on factors like payer type, denial reasons, and outstanding amounts. This segmentation will guide your strategy by allowing you to address different account groups effectively.

4. **Allocate Resources:** Assign appropriate staff members or teams to handle different segments of old AR accounts. Ensure they have the necessary tools, training, and time to focus on recovery.

5. **Set Realistic Timelines:** Establish timelines for each phase of your recovery strategy, from initial contact to resolution. Ensure these timelines are achievable and align with your practice's capacity.

6. **Prioritize High-Impact Accounts:** Focus on accounts with the highest potential for recovery and impact on your practice's financial health. Prioritize those with large outstanding amounts or recurring denial issues.

7. **Create a Workflow Framework:** Develop a structured workflow for your recovery process. Define the steps from account assessment and follow-up to resolution and payment collection.

8. **Implement an Account Tracking System:** Utilize a tracking system or software to monitor the progress of each account. This helps prevent accounts from falling through the cracks and ensures consistent follow-up.

9. **Leverage Multichannel Communication:** Reach out to payers through various communication channels, including phone calls, emails, and formal letters. Different channels can yield different response rates.

10. **Craft Customized Recovery Strategies:** Tailor your recovery approach to each segment of accounts. Consider payer-specific requirements, denial patterns, and past communication history.

11. **Collaborate with Payers:** Engage in constructive conversations with payers to discuss denial reasons and seek resolution. Build relationships with payer representatives to facilitate smoother negotiations.

12. **Utilize Automated Reminders:** Implement automated reminders for follow-up activities to ensure timely actions on accounts. This prevents missed opportunities and maximizes your recovery efforts.

13. **Monitor Progress Regularly:** Hold regular progress review meetings to assess the

effectiveness of your recovery strategy. Adjust your approach based on feedback and results.

14. **Document Communication:** Maintain detailed records of all communication with payers, including dates, times, and content. This documentation can be crucial for appeal submissions and tracking progress.

15. **Review and Revise:** Continuously review your recovery strategy's performance against set goals. Adjust your tactics based on outcomes, keeping in mind the evolving landscape of medical billing.

16. **Ensure Compliance:** Stay up to date with industry regulations and guidelines during your recovery efforts. Compliance is essential to avoid legal issues while pursuing account resolutions.

17. **Team Collaboration:** Foster collaboration among different departments involved in the recovery process, such as billing, coding, and administrative teams. Shared insights can lead to more effective strategies.

18. **Provide Training and Support:** Offer training sessions to your recovery team on negotiation skills, effective communication, and payer-specific protocols. Support their growth and development in this role.

19. **Celebrate Milestones:** Acknowledge and celebrate achievements within your recovery strategy, whether it's a successful negotiation, an account resolved, or a notable reduction in AR aging.

20. **Continuous Improvement Culture:** Encourage your recovery team to provide feedback and insights on the strategy's strengths and areas for improvement. Maintain a culture of learning and

adaptability.

Building an effective recovery strategy requires careful planning, execution, and continuous refinement. By implementing these action items, you'll be better equipped to navigate the complexities of old AR recovery and achieve your practice's financial goals.

EFFECTIVE COMMUNICATION WITH PAYERS

UNLOCKING THE MYSTERIES OF PAYER INTERACTION

In the realm of revenue recovery, effective communication with payers is a spellbinding art—a dance of words and strategies that can transform claim denials into triumphant reimbursements. As we delve into the arcane secrets of this domain, let us harness the wisdom of the Revenue Recovery Wizards to unravel the mysteries and forge a path to financial prosperity.

CRAFTING COMPELLING APPEALS AND RESUBMISSIONS

Behold, the scrolls of appeal and resubmission—a potent duo that holds the key to reclaiming denied claims from the shadows. To wield them effectively is to transmute denial into victory.

The Art of Eloquent Appeal

Like a masterful incantation, craft appeals that weave a compelling narrative, highlighting the medical necessity of the services provided. Harness the power of precise language, detailing the patient's condition, treatment plan, and the alignment with payer guidelines. Each word shall resonate with the payer's heart, urging reconsideration.

The Phoenix's Resurrection

Resubmission, a phoenix rising from the ashes of denial, bears the promise of redemption. Study denial trends and rework the claim with meticulous attention to detail. Amend inaccuracies, furnish missing information, and enhance documentation to ensure a potent claim that emerges stronger than before.

LEVERAGING NEGOTIATION TECHNIQUES FOR HIGHER REIMBURSEMENT

In the grand tapestry of revenue recovery, negotiation is the thread that weaves the fabric of equitable reimbursement. To master this art is to transmute negotiations into treasures untold.

The Enchantment of Preparedness

Before entering negotiations, channel the wisdom of preparation. Delve into payer policies, industry benchmarks, and the specifics of the denied claim. Armed with knowledge, engage in negotiations from a position of strength, presenting your case with confidence.

The Dance of Persuasion

As you negotiate, embrace the dance of persuasion—a delicate interplay of reason, persistence, and charm. Present a compelling argument, backed by evidence and aligned with regulatory guidelines. Navigate the negotiation labyrinth with finesse, ensuring the payer understands the value of your claim.

The Mirror of Compromise

Gaze into the Mirror of Compromise, reflecting the art of finding the middle ground. While advocating for optimal reimbursement, be open to reasonable concessions that lead to a harmonious resolution. This balance shall foster a positive relationship, paving the way for future collaborations.

As you embark on the quest of effective payer communication, remember that each appeal, resubmission, and negotiation is a stroke of the wand—an opportunity to conjure financial restoration from the depths of claim denials. With the wisdom of eloquent appeals and the finesse of negotiation techniques, you shall wield the powers of effective communication, transforming denied claims into the currency of your practice's success.

ACTION ITEMS

1. **Gather Payer Information:** Compile accurate contact details and relevant information for each payer. This includes dedicated phone numbers, email addresses, and preferred modes of

communication.

2. **Craft Compelling Appeal Letters:** Develop template appeal letters that address common denial reasons. Customize these templates for each payer, highlighting relevant details and focusing on concise and persuasive language.

3. **Prepare Clear Resubmission Documentation:** Ensure resubmission documentation is thorough, organized, and includes any additional information requested by the payer. Clearly explain the medical necessity and value of the provided services.

4. **Utilize Negotiation Techniques:** Train your team in negotiation strategies, such as emphasizing the value of the services, proposing win-win solutions, and demonstrating willingness to cooperate for a resolution.

5. **Follow-Up Methodically:** Establish a systematic follow-up schedule with payers after submitting appeals or resubmissions. Consistently track responses, dates of contact, and any agreed-upon actions.

6. **Document All Interactions:** Maintain detailed records of all communications with payers, including call logs, emails, and letters. This documentation helps track progress and provides evidence in case of disputes.

7. **Build Relationships with Payer Representatives:** Establish and nurture positive relationships with payer representatives. Develop a rapport based on professionalism, cooperation, and a shared goal of resolving claims.

8. **Escalate When Necessary:** Have a clear escalation process in place for cases that require higher-level intervention. Know when to involve

supervisors or managers to expedite resolutions.

9. **Leverage Multichannel Communication:** Use various communication channels, such as phone calls, emails, and fax, based on payer preferences. Different payers might respond better to different methods.

10. **Incorporate Appeals Language:** Ensure your appeal letters use language that aligns with the payer's specific policies and requirements. Address their concerns while advocating for the reimbursement of services.

11. **Highlight Medical Necessity:** Emphasize the medical necessity and value of the provided services in your communication. Clearly explain how the services align with the patient's condition and overall treatment plan.

12. **Conduct Training Workshops:** Hold training sessions for your team to improve communication skills, negotiation techniques, and conflict resolution strategies when dealing with payers.

13. **Stay Informed on Payer Policies:** Regularly review payer policies and guidelines to stay updated on any changes that could affect your communication and negotiation strategies.

14. **Analyze Response Patterns:** Analyze patterns in payer responses to appeals and resubmissions. Use this information to refine your communication tactics and tailor your approach to each payer.

15. **Monitor Denial Trends:** Identify common denial trends and address them proactively in your communication. This demonstrates your commitment to continuous improvement and accurate billing.

16. **Implement Time-Sensitive Approaches:** Be aware of deadlines for appeals and resubmissions, and structure your communication to reflect the urgency of the situation while maintaining professionalism.

17. **Seek Feedback from Payers:** After successful appeals or favorable resolutions, seek feedback from payer representatives. Understand what aspects of your communication were effective and use this insight for future interactions.

18. **Role Play Scenarios:** Conduct role-playing exercises where team members simulate interactions with payers. This practice helps refine communication skills and adapt to different payer personalities.

19. **Celebrate Successful Resolutions:** Celebrate and acknowledge successful appeals or negotiated resolutions within your team. Recognize their efforts in effectively communicating with payers to secure reimbursements.

20. **Continuous Learning and Adaptation:** Encourage a culture of continuous learning by sharing success stories, lessons learned, and best practices within your team. Adapt your communication strategies based on evolving payer dynamics.

Effective communication with payers is essential for resolving claim denials and maximizing reimbursements. By implementing these action items, you'll enhance your practice's ability to engage constructively with payers and achieve successful outcomes in the revenue recovery process.

OPTIMIZING CODING AND DOCUMENTATION

UNVEILING THE CODEX OF REVENUE ENHANCEMENT

In the enchanted scrolls of revenue recovery, the chapter on Optimizing Coding and Documentation holds the key to unlocking the hidden treasures of maximum reimbursement. Here, within the labyrinthine corridors of accurate coding and meticulous documentation, we shall unravel the secrets that transform mere claims into golden streams of revenue.

ENSURING CODING ACCURACY AND MEDICAL NECESSITY

The Oracle of Code Mastery

Behold the sacred symbols of medical coding—an intricate language that must be deciphered with precision. The Revenue Recovery Wizards advise meticulous code selection, ensuring each procedure and diagnosis code aligns with the patient's condition and the services rendered. With every code chosen, a portal to rightful reimbursement is opened.

The Quest for Medical Necessity

In the realm of reimbursement, medical necessity is a potent enchantment. Document the patient's condition comprehensively, weaving a narrative that outlines the necessity of the provided services. Align with payer guidelines, illustrating the impact on the patient's health and the broader treatment plan. Through this harmonious alignment, denials are dispelled.

DOCUMENTING SERVICES FOR MAXIMUM REIMBURSEMENT

The Scribe's Mastery

Within the chronicles of documentation lies the power to transcend denials. Capture each element of the patient encounter with meticulous detail—a symphony of notes that resonates with payer expectations. Describe the services rendered, the patient's response, and the provider's expertise, leaving no corner unilluminated.

The Art of Specificity

As you weave the tale of services provided, invoke the spirits of specificity. Record not only what was done but why, delving into the nuances that differentiate levels of care. Illuminate the unique aspects of each patient's journey, ensuring the documentation echoes the richness of the encounter.

The Elixir of Clarity

Let the elixir of clarity flow through your documentation, dispelling ambiguity and uncertainty. Translate medical jargon into patient-friendly language, allowing both payer and patient to comprehend the journey of care. Your documentation shall stand as a beacon of transparency, guiding the path to rightful reimbursement.

In the labyrinthine passages of coding accuracy and the sacred scrolls of documentation, the Revenue Recovery Wizards impart their ancient wisdom. With each accurately chosen code and each meticulously documented encounter, you forge a pathway to maximize reimbursement. As you tread upon this sacred ground, remember that every code and every word is a stroke of your wand, transforming claims into the gold of your practice's prosperity.

ACTION ITEMS

1. **Educate Coding Team:** To ensure accuracy and compliance, provide ongoing training to your coding team about the latest coding guidelines, including CPT, ICD-10, and HCPCS Level II

codes.

2. **Use Clear Documentation Templates:** Develop standardized documentation templates that guide providers in capturing detailed and necessary information for each patient encounter.

3. **Implement Regular Audits:** Conduct routine audits of coded claims to identify any discrepancies or errors. Use this feedback to improve coding accuracy and documentation practices.

4. **Ensure Consistency in Code Assignment:** Implement protocols to ensure consistency in code assignment across different coders, avoiding discrepancies and potential claim denials.

5. **Stay Informed about Regulations:** Keep abreast of evolving regulations, especially those related to medical necessity and coding specificity, and educate your team accordingly.

6. **Focus on Medical Necessity:** Train providers to document the medical necessity of services clearly, outlining the condition being treated and the rationale for the chosen treatment.

7. **Utilize Modifier Codes Appropriately:** Ensure accurate usage of modifier codes when applicable, indicating specific circumstances that warrant additional reimbursement.

8. **Collaborate with Providers:** Foster collaboration between coders and providers to clarify any coding-related questions and ensure accurate representation of services provided.

9. **Regularly Update Codebooks:** Keep your coding resources and codebooks up to date with the latest code changes and revisions.

10. **Leverage EHR Functionality:** Utilize electronic

health record (EHR) system features to streamline coding processes and ensure documentation aligns with coding requirements.

11. **Document Changes and Corrections:** Implement a protocol for documenting any changes or corrections made to codes and documentation after initial submission.

12. **Address Documentation Insufficiencies:** Proactively address any documentation insufficiencies with providers to prevent claim denials due to incomplete or ambiguous documentation.

13. **Provide Regular Feedback:** Establish a feedback loop between coders and providers, sharing instances where improved documentation could lead to more accurate coding and claim success.

14. **Implement Coding Guidelines:** Create a comprehensive coding guideline document that outlines coding conventions and specific instructions for various scenarios.

15. **Review Payer Policies:** Understand the coding and documentation requirements of different payers and tailor your practices accordingly to reduce claim denials.

16. **Double-Check Commonly Denied Codes:** Identify frequently denied codes and ensure that documentation provides ample justification for the use of these codes.

17. **Engage Coding Specialists:** If necessary, consider engaging certified coding specialists who have expertise in complex coding scenarios, reducing the risk of coding-related denials.

18. **Monitor Industry Updates:** Stay updated with

industry news and updates related to coding and documentation practices, adjusting your strategies as needed.

19. **Document Best Practices:** Create a repository of coding and documentation of best practices, enabling your team to refer to proven methods when facing specific challenges.

By implementing these action items, you'll enhance your coding and documentation practices, leading to accurate claims, reduced denials, and improved reimbursement rates.

NAVIGATING THE APPEALS PROCESS

UNVEILING THE ART OF APPEAL CONJURATION

In the enchanted realm of revenue recovery, the chapter of Navigating the Appeals Process unveils the arcane art of reclaiming denied claims. As we embark on this mystical journey, you shall acquire the knowledge and strategies to wield the magic of appeals, turning the tides of denial into the currents of reimbursement.

UNDERSTANDING THE APPEALS TIMELINE AND PROCEDURES

The Chronicles of Denial

The saga of denied claims unveils itself in a series of stages, each with its own temporal rhythm. Delve into the sacred scrolls of payer communication, uncovering the timeline within which appeals must be summoned. The Revenue Recovery Wizards shall guide you through this temporal dance, ensuring your appeals are summoned with precision.

The Dance of Documentation

Prepare thy arsenal of supporting documentation—a symphony of evidence that echoes the necessity and legitimacy of your claim. Understand the intricacies of the appeals submission process, as each scroll and enchantment must be adhered to. Allow the wisdom of the wizards to illuminate the path, ensuring your appeal speaks with resounding clarity.

STRATEGIES FOR SUCCESSFUL CLAIM APPEALS

The Emissaries of Persuasion

Enlist the support of persuasive enchantments in your appeal missives. Craft a narrative that not only presents the case for reimbursement but compels the payer to reconsider their initial judgment. The wizards advise invoking empathy and presenting the patient's journey as a tapestry of necessity, woven with the threads of compassionate care.

The Alchemy of Evidence

Within your appeal, the alchemical blend of evidence shall work its magic. Present medical records, documentation, and expert opinions that support your cause. The Revenue Recovery Wizards remind you to harmonize these elements into a symphony of validation, leaving no doubt of the justness of your plea.

The Confluence of Compliance

Align your appeal with the cosmic currents of payer guidelines and regulations. Engage in the rituals of compliance, ensuring your appeal adheres to the payer's expectations. The wizards' counsel urges you to navigate this maze with precision, transforming compliance into a wand that bends the tides of appeal in your favor.

As you traverse the labyrinthine passages of the appeals process, the Revenue Recovery Wizards shall illuminate your path. With each scroll you write and each piece of evidence you present, you wield the magic of appeal conjuration. Denied claims shall quiver in the face of your incantations, their denials transformed into the echoes of reimbursement.

ACTION ITEMS

1. **Understand Payer Appeal Guidelines:** Familiarize yourself with each payer's appeal guidelines, timelines, and submission procedures to ensure compliance and maximize your chances of success.

2. **Create an Appeals Calendar:** Establish a centralized calendar that tracks appeal deadlines for different payers, helping you avoid missed opportunities for resubmission.

3. **Categorize Denials:** Classify denials based on common reasons (e.g., coding errors and documentation deficiencies) to streamline your appeal process and identify recurring issues.

4. **Gather Comprehensive Information:** Collect all relevant documentation, including medical records, claims, coding documentation, and any correspondence with the payer, before initiating an appeal.

5. **Craft Persuasive Appeal Letters:** Develop well-structured appeal letters that clearly outline the reason for the appeal, provide supporting evidence, and present a strong case for reconsideration.

6. **Include Supporting Documentation:** Attach all necessary supporting documentation, such as medical records, diagnostic reports, and any additional information that strengthens your appeal.

7. **Engage Clinical Experts:** Consult with clinical experts within your organization to provide insights and medical justifications for denied claims, especially when dealing with medical necessity disputes.

8. **Review Payer Policies:** Scrutinize payer policies to identify discrepancies or misinterpretations that may have led to the denial, enabling you to address these points in your appeal.

9. **Emphasize Corrective Measures:** Outline the corrective actions you've taken to address the issues that led to the denial, demonstrating your commitment to compliance and improvement.

10. **Submit Appeals Promptly:** Adhere to the specified appeal timelines to avoid missing your chance to challenge the denial. Submit appeals promptly to increase the likelihood of success.

11. **Track Appeal Progress:** Maintain a systematic tracking system to monitor the progress of each

appeal, ensuring timely follow-ups and preventing any appeals from falling through the cracks.

12. **Utilize Online Portals:** If available, utilize online portals provided by payers to streamline the appeal submission process, ensuring accurate and efficient communication.

13. **Engage with Payer Representatives:** Establish open lines of communication with payer representatives, engaging in dialogue to better understand the reasons for the denial and negotiate favorable resolutions.

14. **Escalate if Necessary:** If initial appeal efforts are unsuccessful, escalate the appeal to the next level within the payer's hierarchy, engaging higher-level representatives if needed.

15. **Document Each Step:** Maintain a detailed record of your appeal process, including communication logs, submission dates, and outcomes, to facilitate accountability and future reference.

16. **Analyze Appeal Outcomes:** Regularly review the outcomes of your appeal efforts to identify patterns and areas for improvement in your claims and documentation practices.

17. **Consider External Support:** If faced with complex or recurring denials, consider consulting with external experts or legal counsel experienced in payer appeals to bolster your case.

18. **Benchmark Appeal Success:** Keep track of your appeal success rates, benchmarking them against industry standards to gauge the effectiveness of your appeal strategies.

19. **Share Learnings:** Disseminate lessons learned from successful appeals to your team, promoting

continuous improvement in coding, documentation, and appeal strategies.

20. **Seek Feedback from Payers:** Request feedback from payers on denied claims to better understand their reasoning and identify opportunities to align your processes with payer expectations.

By implementing these action items, you'll enhance your ability to navigate the appeals process effectively, increase your chances of overturning denials, and ultimately improve your revenue recovery efforts.

OUR REAL MOTIVE FOR WRITING THIS BOOK

By this point you might be wondering why we're spilling all these magical secrets at such a humble price. There's a deeper purpose behind it all – a purpose that goes beyond just the mystical realm of billing and insurance tricks.

You see, our heart's quest is to combat the shadowy opioid crisis that's been casting a dark cloud over our society. Our focus? Well, it's fixated on aiding those brave souls working in behavioral health and substance use centers. We're all about enabling them to weave their healing spells and provide as much treatment as humanly possible.

To make that happen, these centers need to summon forth the gold, in the form of insurance company payments, Medicaid blessings, and Medicare charms. The more coins they collect from these sources, the less they have to ask their patients to dig into their pockets – those very pockets that might be clinging on to hope while battling the grip of substances.

We've gazed into the abyss and witnessed firsthand the havoc that substance use wrecks upon families, friends, and cherished ones. If we can aid these providers in guiding their patients toward the path of substance-free existence, then we reckon we've done our part. Yet, for our enchanted quest to reach its zenith, we need your conjuring touch. Yes, we're summoning your assistance.

Now, we're about to ask something quite grand of you... If this tome has already begun to weave its enchantment upon you, and you've found the secrets within its pages to be worth their weight in gold, it'd be an act of magic if you could kindly spread the word. Extend your wand of goodwill to those fellow providers who stand shoulder to shoulder with you in weaving the tapestry of exceptional patient care. All we request is a mere moment of your precious time – to inscribe an honest review, like an incantation that echoes through the digital realms.

We recognize that time is a precious gem in the treasure chest of life. And that's exactly why we've poured our very essence into this book – to ensure it's a trove of wisdom worthy of your investment. Your review, dear conjurer, holds immense power. It's a guiding light for other providers, leading them to the secrets contained within and helping them discern whether this magical tome is the real deal.

But, of course, the wand of choice is yours. When you're ready, journey to the Amazon realm and seek out the shimmering words, "Review this product." With a mere flick of your virtual quill, you'll weave your words into the tapestry of reviews. It's as simple as a wave of the hand.

With hearts brimming with gratitude, we thank you from the deepest caverns of our enchanted realm. It's spirited providers like you who fuel our magical endeavors.

And now, without further ado, let's plunge back into the mystical world of wizardry that lies within these pages.

NEGOTIATION STRATEGIES FOR RECOVERY

HARNESSING THE ART OF PAYER PARLEY

Within the realm of revenue recovery, the chapter of Negotiation Strategies for Recovery reveals the ancient art of parley with payers. As you embark on this journey, you shall acquire the wisdom and techniques to wield negotiation as a potent enchantment, bending the currents of reimbursement to your will.

NEGOTIATING WITH PAYERS FOR FAVORABLE OUTCOMES

The Envoys of Reimbursement

Step into the arena of negotiation with a demeanor of confidence and mastery. The wizards shall impart upon you the essence of assertive diplomacy, ensuring your presence commands respect from the payer realm. Through words and manner, convey that you are a sorcerer of value, conjuring revenue that rightfully belongs to your practice.

The Dance of Compromise

Engage in the art of compromise, where the melodies of give and take weave the tapestry of favorable outcomes. Delve into the arcane rituals of finding common ground, allowing the Revenue Recovery Wizards to guide you in the delicate choreography of negotiation. Embrace the magic of give and receive, and watch as reimbursement barriers crumble beneath your skillful steps.

TECHNIQUES TO OVERCOME REIMBURSEMENT BARRIERS

The Mirror of Evidence

Reflect the payer's gaze upon the mirror of evidence. With clarity and precision, present the strengths of your claim, showcasing the value and necessity of the services rendered. The wizards advise adorning your argument with gems of data and statistics, turning the tides of negotiation in your favor.

The Enchantment of Persistence

Be a steadfast enchantress or enchanter, holding firm in your pursuit of favorable terms. The Revenue Recovery Wizards counsel you to stand resolute in the face of challenges, for the path to reimbursement is often paved with determination. With each negotiation, your skills shall evolve, and your results shall flourish.

The Spell of Creative Solutions

Weave a spell of innovative solutions that transcend the mundane. Unlock the potential of alternative arrangements and payment structures, revealing to payers the hidden avenues of collaboration. The wizards' guidance shall help you craft offers that harmonize with the payer's desires, unlocking the vaults of reimbursement.

In the realm of negotiation, you become a maestro of revenue orchestration, directing the melodies of dialogue to your advantage. The Revenue Recovery Wizards bestow upon you the gifts of confidence, diplomacy, and strategic finesse, allowing you to engage in negotiation as a true conjurer of reimbursement. As you traverse the landscape of payer parley, envision each negotiation as a dance of power, with you as the choreographer, leading the way to favorable outcomes and ensuring the financial prosperity of your practice.

ACTION ITEMS

1. **Analyze Payer Contracts:** Thoroughly review payer contracts to understand negotiated reimbursement rates, fee schedules, and any clauses related to appeals and negotiations.

2. **Gather Data and Evidence:** Collect data on industry-standard reimbursement rates and gather evidence of your practice's performance, patient outcomes, and value delivered.

3. **Know Your Worth:** Understand the value your practice brings to the payer, highlighting quality of care, patient satisfaction, and any unique services or specialties offered.

4. **Prepare Compelling Arguments:** Develop persuasive arguments that emphasize your practice's strengths and why your reimbursement rates should be increased or adjusted.

5. **Identify Payer Motivations:** Research the payer's motivations, challenges, and strategic goals to tailor your negotiation approach accordingly.

6. **Leverage Comparative Data:** Present comparative data from similar practices or industry benchmarks to support your request for better reimbursement rates.

7. **Highlight Unique Value Propositions:** Showcase any distinctive services, outcomes, or patient satisfaction scores that set your practice apart and justify higher reimbursement.

8. **Demonstrate Cost-Effectiveness:** Illustrate how your practice's services contribute to cost savings for the payer by reducing hospital readmissions or unnecessary procedures.

9. **Package Services Strategically:** Bundle services or procedures to create appealing packages that offer value to payers while also justifying higher reimbursement.

10. **Showcase Quality Metrics:** Present quality metrics and performance indicators that demonstrate your practice's commitment to delivering high-quality care and positive patient outcomes.

11. **Engage in Constructive Dialogue:** Initiate open and respectful discussions with payer representatives, aiming to find common ground and mutually beneficial solutions.

12. **Negotiate Long-Term Contracts:** Consider

negotiating longer-term contracts that provide stability and predictability to both parties, potentially leading to improved reimbursement terms.

13. **Articulate the Patient Experience:** Share patient testimonials and stories that highlight the positive impact of your practice's care on patient lives.

14. **Be Patient and Persistent:** Negotiations can take time. Be patient and persistent in your efforts, maintaining a professional and respectful demeanor throughout the process.

15. **Utilize Data Analytics:** Utilize data analytics tools to present data-driven insights that showcase your practice's performance and its correlation with improved reimbursement.

16. **Offer Performance Guarantees:** If appropriate, consider offering performance guarantees tied to specific outcomes or quality metrics as part of your negotiation.

17. **Highlight Market Share:** Emphasize your practice's market share and patient volume as evidence of your contribution to the payer's network.

18. **Demonstrate ROI:** Present a clear return on investment (ROI) by showcasing how increased reimbursement rates align with improved patient outcomes and practice growth.

19. **Negotiate from a Position of Strength:** Leverage your practice's strengths, such as specialized services, patient demand, or reputation, to negotiate from a position of strength.

20. **Seek Win-Win Solutions:** Aim for win-win outcomes that benefit both parties, recognizing

that a positive relationship with payers can yield long-term advantages.

By implementing these action items, you'll be better equipped to navigate negotiations with payers, strategically advocate for fair reimbursement rates, and optimize your practice's revenue recovery efforts.

TRACKING AND MONITORING RECOVERY PROGRESS

UNVEILING THE OBSERVATORY OF PROSPERITY

As your journey through the realm of old accounts receivable recovery continues, you now stand at the threshold of the chapter on Tracking and Monitoring Recovery Progress. Here, the path widens, revealing the panoramic vista of the Observatory of Prosperity—a place where the stars of data and analytics align to guide your practice toward the shores of financial success.

Implementing Effective Reporting and Analytics

The Seer's Crystal Ball

Enter the chamber of effective reporting and analytics,

where data unveils its hidden truths. The wizards impart upon you the art of crafting insightful reports that illuminate the path of recovery. With each glance into the seer's crystal ball of data, you gain clarity on the currents of reimbursement, identifying patterns, trends, and opportunities.

The Alchemy of Data Interpretation

Transform raw data into the gold of actionable insights. The wizards' wisdom guides you in deciphering the language of numbers, translating them into meaningful narratives. Learn to extract gems of knowledge from the caverns of data, refining your strategies and directing your recovery efforts with precision.

Making Informed Decisions Based on Recovery Data

The Council of Strategy

Assemble the council of strategy, where data-driven decisions shape the destiny of your practice. The Revenue Recovery Wizards advocate for informed deliberations, where the insights gleaned from recovery data influence the choices you make. Envision yourself as a sage ruler, consulting the stars of analytics to guide your every move.

The Navigator's Compass

Allow recovery data to become your trusty compass, steering your practice through the turbulent seas of revenue recovery. The wizards advise you to adjust your course based on the signals received from the celestial tapestry of data. With each adjustment, you draw nearer to the shores of optimal reimbursement.

The Cauldron of Continuous Improvement

Stir the cauldron of continuous improvement, infusing your practice with the elixir of data-enhanced progress. The wizards' spell encourages you to embrace the iterative nature of recovery, using data as a potion to refine your strategies, enhance your approaches, and ultimately fortify your revenue cycle.

In the Observatory of Prosperity, you ascend to new heights of financial prowess, harnessing the powers of data and analytics to illuminate your path. As you implement effective reporting, interpret data, and make informed decisions, you metamorphose into a skilled astronomer of revenue recovery.

The Revenue Recovery Wizards empower you to wield the tools of insight and wisdom, allowing you to navigate the constellations of reimbursement with confidence and precision. As you gaze upon the stars of data, remember that each point of light holds a key to your practice's financial prosperity, guiding you toward the realization of your revenue recovery aspirations.

ACTION ITEMS

1. **Define Key Performance Indicators (KPIs):** Identify and define the KPIs that align with your recovery goals, such as claim acceptance rates, denial rates, reimbursement amounts, and average time to resolution.

2. **Select Relevant Metrics:** Choose metrics that provide actionable insights into different stages of

the recovery process, from claim submission to successful reimbursement.

3. **Implement Data Collection Tools:** Utilize practice management software or specialized tools to automatically collect and track relevant data points, ensuring accuracy and consistency.

4. **Establish Reporting Intervals:** Set regular reporting intervals, whether daily, weekly, or monthly, to monitor progress and identify trends over time.

5. **Create Visual Dashboards:** Develop visual dashboards or reports that provide a clear snapshot of your recovery progress, making it easier to identify areas needing improvement.

6. **Analyze Denial Patterns:** Regularly analyze denial patterns to pinpoint recurring issues and address root causes that hinder successful recovery.

7. **Compare Performance to Targets:** Continuously compare actual performance against established targets and benchmarks to assess your practice's recovery effectiveness.

8. **Identify Bottlenecks:** Identify bottlenecks or delays in the recovery process by analyzing the time taken for each stage, from claim submission to reimbursement.

9. **Segment Data for Analysis:** Segment recovery data by payer, provider, service type, or any other relevant criteria to gain insights into variations and trends.

10. **Engage in Root Cause Analysis:** Perform root cause analysis for recurring denials or delays to determine underlying issues and develop corrective

actions.

11. **Share Data with Teams:** Share recovery progress data with relevant teams or staff members to foster transparency and encourage collaborative problem-solving.

12. **Set Improvement Goals:** Set specific improvement goals based on the insights gained from tracking and monitoring recovery progress.

13. **Implement Continuous Improvement:** Continuously iterate and improve your recovery process based on the data-driven insights obtained.

14. **Benchmark Against Industry Standards:** Compare your recovery progress with industry benchmarks and best practices to identify areas for further enhancement.

15. **Use Predictive Analytics:** Implement predictive analytics to forecast potential bottlenecks or issues in the recovery process, allowing proactive intervention.

16. **Identify High-Value Accounts:** Identify high-value accounts with larger reimbursement potential and prioritize efforts accordingly.

17. **Implement Automated Alerts:** Set up automated alerts or notifications for key performance thresholds, enabling prompt action when deviations occur.

18. **Celebrate Milestones**: Celebrate milestones and achievements in recovery progress, motivating your team and fostering a positive working environment.

19. **Review Process Efficiency:** Regularly review the efficiency of your recovery process, identifying opportunities to streamline and expedite certain

stages.

20. **Feedback and Adaptation:** Encourage feedback
from team members involved in the recovery
process, using their insights to adapt and refine
your monitoring strategy.

By implementing these action items, you'll establish a
robust system for tracking and monitoring the progress of
your recovery efforts. This data-driven approach will help
you identify areas for improvement, optimize your
recovery process, and achieve your revenue recovery goals
more effectively.

DIY TOOLS FOR OLD AR RECOVERY

HARNESSING THE ARTIFACTS OF EMPOWERMENT

In this enchanted trove of knowledge, we unveil the DIY Tools for Old AR Recovery, a collection of artifacts that will empower you to wield the magic of recovery with your own hands. As you traverse this chapter, you'll discover a cache of tools designed to equip you for the journey ahead, each imbued with the potential to transform challenges into triumphs.

CLAIM DENIAL TROUBLESHOOTING CHECKLIST

The Oracle's Scroll

Unveil the Claim Denial Troubleshooting Checklist, a

sacred scroll etched with incantations to decipher the enigma of denials. This mystical document guides you through a labyrinth of questions and prompts, illuminating the root causes of claim denials. With each query, you unveil the secrets hidden within the depths of your unpaid claims, revealing the keys to resolution.

The "Claim Denial Troubleshooting Checklist" is designed to help you systematically identify and address issues leading to claim denials. This checklist will assist you in thoroughly reviewing denied claims and taking the necessary steps to rectify the situation. Here's an example of what the checklist might look like:

Account Information

☑ Verify patient information (name, date of birth, insurance details) for accuracy.

☑ Confirm that the patient's insurance coverage was active on the date of service.

☑ Check if the patient's policy number and group number were correctly entered.

Coding and Documentation

☑ Review the coding for accuracy, including CPT codes and diagnosis codes.

☑ Ensure that the services provided match the codes billed.

☑ Confirm that the documentation supports medical necessity for the services rendered.

Submission Errors

☑ Check for any technical errors in claim submission, such

as missing fields or formatting issues.

☑ Validate that the claim was submitted within the payer's designated timeframe.

☑ Verify that the claim was sent to the correct payer and billing address.

Claim Rejections

☑ Identify the reason for rejection (e.g., duplicate claim, missing information, invalid procedure code).

☑ Address the specific rejection reason as indicated by the payer.

Prior Authorization

☑ Verify if the services rendered required prior authorization.

☑ Confirm that the necessary prior authorization was obtained before providing services.

Coordination of Benefits

☑ Determine if the patient has other insurance coverage that needs to be coordinated.

☑ Ensure that primary and secondary insurance information is accurate and up to date.

Appeal Opportunities

☑ Identify whether the claim denial can be appealed.

☑ Review payer guidelines for appeal procedures and timeframes.

Documentation of Communication

☑ Keep records of all communication with payers regarding the denial.

☑ Document dates, names of individuals spoken to, and details of conversations.

Internal Review

☑ Conduct an internal review to prevent similar denials in the future.

☑ Implement corrective actions based on the findings of the review.

Follow-up and Resolution

☑ Resubmit corrected claims with necessary documentation and coding.

☑ Track the progress of resubmitted claims to ensure timely processing.

Analysis and Reporting

☑ Analyze trends in claim denials to identify common patterns.

☑ Generate reports to monitor denial rates and track improvements over time.

This checklist serves as a comprehensive guide to systematically troubleshoot denied claims and take corrective actions. By following these steps, you'll be better equipped to address claim denials efficiently and minimize their impact on your revenue cycle. Remember to customize the checklist based on your specific practice's needs and workflows.

SAMPLE APPEAL LETTERS AND TEMPLATES

The Quill of Persuasion

Command the Quill of Persuasion, a mystical writing tool that conjures eloquent words of appeal. Within its ink lies the power to craft compelling appeal letters and templates, each sentence resonating with the magic of persuasion. Let your appeals soar on the wings of this enchanted quill, capturing the attention of payers and guiding them toward favorable outcomes.

When faced with claim denials, a well-crafted appeal letter can make all the difference in getting your claim successfully reconsidered and approved. Below are some sample appeal letter templates you can use as a starting point. Remember to tailor these templates to your specific situation and provide accurate details.

Medical Necessity Appeal

[Your Name]

[Your Title]

[Your Medical Practice Name]

[Your Address]

[City, State, ZIP]

[Date]

[Insurance Company Name]

[Claims Department]

[Address]

[City, State, ZIP]

Re: Appeal of Claim Denial [Patient Name], [Claim Number]

Dear [Insurance Company Name] Claims Department,

I am writing to appeal the denial of the claim for [Patient Name], which was submitted under claim number [Claim Number]. The denial states that the procedure [Procedure Code] was not considered medically necessary.

I strongly disagree with this decision as [Patient Name]'s condition and medical history warrant the procedure in question. [Provide a detailed explanation of the medical necessity, patient's history, and any relevant supporting documentation.]

I kindly request a thorough review of this appeal and urge

you to reconsider your decision. Please find attached the necessary medical records and documentation supporting the medical necessity of this procedure.

Thank you for your prompt attention to this matter. I look forward to a favorable resolution.

Sincerely,

[Your Name]

[Your Title]

[Email Address]

[Phone Number]

[Fax Number]

Coding Error Appeal

[Your Name]

[Your Title]

[Your Medical Practice Name]

[Your Address]

[City, State, ZIP]

[Date]

[Insurance Company Name]

[Claims Department]

[Address]

[City, State, ZIP]

Re: Appeal of Claim Denial [Patient Name], [Claim Number]

Dear [Insurance Company Name] Claims Department,

I am writing to appeal the denial of the claim for [Patient Name], which was submitted under claim number [Claim Number]. The denial is based on an alleged coding error with procedure code [Procedure Code].

After a thorough review of the claim and medical documentation, I believe the coding error is unfounded. The procedure performed was accurately coded, and I have attached the relevant medical records to support this assertion.

I kindly request that you reconsider your decision and review the attached documentation. Your prompt attention to this matter is greatly appreciated.

Sincerely,

[Your Name]

[Your Title]

[Email Address]

[Phone Number]

[Fax Number]

Feel free to modify and expand these templates based on your specific needs and the type of appeal you are making. Remember to include any relevant documentation and provide accurate details to increase the chances of a successful appeal.

Please note that the above templates are just examples. It's important to customize them according to your practice's details and the specifics of each claim denial situation.

CLAIMS AUDIT WORKSHEET AND ACTION PLAN

The Map of Clarity

Unroll the Claims Audit Worksheet and Action Plan, a map to guide you through the labyrinth of claims assessment. With this tool in hand, you embark on a quest to scrutinize the fabric of your claims, identifying patterns, discrepancies, and opportunities. As you fill the worksheet with insights, you weave an action plan that leads you toward optimized reimbursement.

The Wand of Resolution

Inscribe your action plan with the Wand of Resolution, a tool of empowerment that channels your intent into actionable steps. Wave this wand and watch as it transforms your observations into strategies, your insights into actions. With a flick of the wrist, you initiate the cascade of changes that will elevate your practice's recovery journey.

As part of your Old Accounts Receivable Recovery process, conducting a comprehensive claims audit can help identify areas of improvement and prioritize your recovery efforts. Use the following Claims Audit Worksheet to systematically review and assess your denied or unpaid claims.

Claims Audit Worksheet

Claim Information

Claim Number

Date of Service

Patient Name

Payer Name

Reason for Denial

Denial Code

Explanation of Denial

Claim Details

Procedure Code(s)

Service Units/Quantity

Diagnosis Code(s)

Total Charged Amount

Supporting Documentation

Attach any relevant medical records, notes, and other supporting documentation related to the claim.

Review Process

Was the claim submitted accurately?

Were the correct procedure and diagnosis codes used?

Was medical necessity adequately documented?

Possible Errors or Issues

Identify any errors, discrepancies, or gaps in documentation that may have contributed to the denial.

Root Cause Analysis

What caused the denial? Was it a coding error, lack of medical necessity documentation, coordination of benefits issue, or another reason?

Action Plan

Outline the steps to rectify the denial and reprocess the claim.

Assign responsibilities for each step.

Set a timeline for resolution.

Action Plan

Step 1: Rectify Errors: Correct any coding errors or inaccuracies in the claim.

Step 2: Gather Documentation: Collect any missing or additional documentation required to support the claim.

Step 3: Resubmission: Update the claim with accurate information and documentation. Submit the corrected claim to the payer.

Step 4: Follow-Up: Monitor the status of the resubmitted claim. Contact the payer for updates if necessary.

Step 5: Appeal: If the claim is denied again, consider the appeal process. Craft a well-documented appeal letter and submit it to the payer.

Step 6: Review Process: Evaluate the root cause of the denial and identify process improvements to prevent similar denials in the future.

By using this Claims Audit Worksheet and Action Plan, you can systematically address denied claims, take corrective actions, and improve your recovery efforts. Remember that consistency and thoroughness are key to achieving a successful Old Accounts Receivable Recovery.

Feel free to modify and expand this worksheet and action plan template based on your practice's needs and preferences. The goal is to create a structured and organized approach to addressing denied claims and improving your revenue recovery process.

As you unlock these DIY tools, you become a practitioner of ancient arts, wielding the artifacts of empowerment to master the craft of old accounts receivable recovery. The knowledge contained within these tools transforms you into a sorcerer of resolution, capable of dispelling denials, crafting appeals, and charting the course toward optimized reimbursement.

With the Claim Denial Troubleshooting Checklist, Sample Appeal Letters and Templates, and the Claims Audit Worksheet and Action Plan at your disposal, you stand ready to embrace the challenges of recovery and emerge victorious in your quest for financial prosperity.

ACTION ITEMS

1. **Claim Denial Troubleshooting Checklist:** Create a comprehensive checklist that guides your team through the process of identifying and addressing common claim denial issues. Include steps to verify patient information, review coding accuracy, check for required documentation, and navigate payer-specific guidelines.

2. **Sample Appeal Letters and Templates:** Develop a library of well-crafted appeal letter templates tailored to different denial reasons. Include placeholders for inserting specific patient and claim details, making customization easier for each case.

3. **Claims Audit Worksheet and Action Plan:** Design a structured claims audit worksheet

that allows your team to systematically review denied claims. Incorporate columns for tracking denial reasons, required actions, responsible parties, and deadlines.

4. **Documentation Improvement Guide:** Create a guide that outlines best practices for accurate and comprehensive documentation to support claim submissions. Include tips on documenting medical necessity, proper coding, and other key elements that impact reimbursement.

5. **Appeal Submission Checklist:** Develop a checklist to ensure all necessary components are included when submitting appeals. List required documents, codes, narratives, and any supporting medical records.

6. **Recovery Progress Tracker:** Design a tracker that monitors the progress of each denied claim from appeal submission to resolution. Include columns for tracking dates, actions taken, communications with payers, and outcomes.

7. **Payer Contact Database:** Create a centralized database with contact information for different payers' customer service and appeals departments. Include notes on preferred communication methods and escalation procedures.

8. **Coding Reference Guide:** Compile a reference guide with common CPT, ICD-10, and HCPCS codes relevant to your practice's specialties. Offer coding tips and cross-reference information to reduce coding errors.

9. **Billing and Reimbursement FAQs:**

Develop a document that answers frequently asked questions related to billing, reimbursement, and claims. Cover topics like insurance verification, patient statements, and common denial reasons.

10. **Denial Reason Analysis Tool:** Build a tool that helps your team analyze denial patterns and trends over time. Create visualizations that highlight the most common denial reasons and the associated financial impact.

11. **Training Videos and Webinars:** Record instructional videos or webinars that guide staff through the process of using DIY tools effectively. Cover topics such as filling out appeal letters, using the claims audit worksheet, and navigating payer portals.

12. **Educational Resources Library:** Curate a library of articles, whitepapers, and resources related to old AR recovery strategies. Provide insights on industry changes, regulatory updates, and best practices.

By offering these DIY tools, you empower your team with resources to enhance their efficiency and effectiveness in tackling old accounts receivable recovery. These tools can be instrumental in streamlining processes, improving communication, and increasing the success rate of your recovery efforts.

WHEN TO SEEK PROFESSIONAL ASSISTANCE

GUIDING STARS ON THE PATH TO MASTERY

Amid the tapestry of old accounts receivable recovery, there may come a time when the heavens themselves whisper that it is wise to seek the aid of cosmic allies. In this chapter, we unveil the celestial signs that indicate your journey could be enhanced by the guidance of medical billing partners—sorcerers who have dedicated their lives to the art of revenue recovery.

SIGNS YOUR RECOVERY EFFORTS NEED EXPERT SUPPORT

The Cosmic Alignments: As you gaze upon the cosmic alignments, take heed of the signs that reveal themselves in your recovery endeavors. Is the constellation of denied claims casting shadows upon your practice's prosperity? Do the stars of confusion and frustration obscure your path? When your efforts yield only a faint glimmer of success, it is a telltale sign that the time has come to seek expert guidance.

The Oracle's Whisper: Listen closely to the oracle's whisper—a subtle intuition that speaks to your heart. When the perplexing labyrinth of claim denials leaves you befuddled, and the complexities of reimbursement threaten to engulf you, the oracle's whisper may nudge you toward the cosmic wisdom of medical billing partners.

HOW MEDICAL BILLING PARTNERS CAN ACCELERATE YOUR RECOVERY

The Guild of Mastery

Envision a guild of mastery, a sacred enclave where medical billing partners gather to share their wisdom. These seasoned sorcerers possess the knowledge and experience to navigate the treacherous currents of revenue recovery. They wield the power of strategy, the spellwork of negotiation, and the artistry of appeals, channeling these forces to bring about the alchemical transformation of denials into reimbursement.

The Elixir of Expertise

The medical billing partners offer an elixir of expertise—a potion that fortifies your practice against the perils of denied claims. They harness the magic of meticulous documentation, ensuring that every claim bears the seal of accuracy and medical necessity. With their guidance, the arcane coding and billing incantations become second nature, and your revenue cycle dances harmoniously with the rhythms of success.

The Cosmic Convergence

As your journey aligns with medical billing partners, you experience a cosmic convergence—a harmonious merging of your purpose with their guidance. Together, you chart a course through the celestial realms of denied claims, utilizing their insights to navigate challenges and seize opportunities. The cosmic forces of recovery flow through you, infusing your practice with newfound vitality.

The Pact of Prosperity

Forge a pact of prosperity with medical billing partners, an unbreakable bond that promises mutual success. Their expertise is your compass, guiding you toward optimized reimbursement and financial well-being. With their support, you transcend the limitations of DIY efforts, embracing the true potential of your practice's revenue recovery.

Embrace the signs, heed the oracle's whisper, and consider the cosmic wisdom of medical billing partners. When your journey through old accounts receivable recovery encounters cosmic crossroads, these allies stand ready to illuminate your path, amplify your efforts, and elevate your practice to new heights of financial prosperity.

ACTION ITEMS

1. **Performance Assessment:** Regularly evaluate your team's success rate in recovering old AR to

identify when your internal efforts might be falling short. Set clear benchmarks for recovery percentages and timelines to gauge performance.

2. **Complex Case Evaluation:** Establish criteria for identifying complex or high-value cases that might require specialized expertise. Implement a review process to determine if certain cases exceed your team's capabilities.

3. **Resource and Workload Analysis:** Monitor your team's workload and assess if they have the capacity to handle an influx of challenging cases without compromising on existing responsibilities.

4. **Financial Impact Assessment:** Calculate the potential financial impact of unresolved old AR and compare it to the cost of hiring professional assistance. Determine the breakeven point where outsourcing becomes a financially prudent option.

5. **Internal Training Evaluation:** Assess the effectiveness of your team's training programs and ongoing education in addressing complex old AR recovery challenges. Identify any gaps in knowledge or skills that might warrant external expertise.

6. **Continuous Denial Patterns:** Keep track of recurring denial patterns that your team struggles to address effectively. If certain denial reasons persist despite your team's efforts, consider seeking professional guidance.

7. **Changing Regulations and Guidelines:** Stay updated on changes in healthcare regulations and payer guidelines that impact AR recovery. If new rules introduce complexities beyond your team's expertise, consider consulting professionals who specialize in the area.

8. **Time Sensitivity and Urgency:** Evaluate whether the urgency of recovering certain old AR cases is hindering your team's ability to focus on other essential tasks. Determine if outsourcing time-sensitive cases can relieve the pressure on your internal resources.

9. **Exploring External Expertise:** Research and identify reputable medical billing partners with proven expertise in old AR recovery. Request consultations or assessments from potential partners to understand how they can enhance your recovery efforts.

10. **Cost-Benefit Analysis:** Conduct a thorough analysis of the potential return on investment (ROI) from hiring professionals for challenging cases. Compare the ROI against the costs of seeking external help to make an informed decision.

11. **Feedback from Team:** Encourage your internal team to provide feedback on cases they believe could benefit from external assistance. Create an open channel for them to express their needs and challenges.

12. **Resource Allocation:** Assess your team's skills, experience, and bandwidth to determine if redirecting their focus from other critical tasks to old AR recovery would be detrimental.

By implementing these action items, you'll be able to effectively gauge when the complexities of old AR recovery warrant seeking professional assistance. Making well-informed decisions based on objective assessments and clear criteria will help you ensure that your recovery efforts remain efficient and effective.

SUCCESS STORIES AND CASE STUDIES

ILLUMINATING THE PATH OF TRIUMPH

Amidst the realm of old accounts receivable recovery, tales of triumphant conquests shine like beacons, guiding practitioners toward the pinnacle of financial success. In this chapter, we unveil a constellation of success stories and case studies—a tapestry woven with threads of perseverance, strategy, and mastery. These luminous examples showcase the power of effective recovery efforts, offering insights, inspiration, and valuable lessons for those embarking on their own journey of revenue reclamation.

REAL-LIFE EXAMPLES OF SUCCESSFUL OLD AR RECOVERY

The Phoenix Rebirth

Witness the tale of a medical practice teetering on the precipice of financial despair, burdened by a constellation of denied claims. Through the guidance of medical billing partners, diligent appeals, and strategic negotiations, this practice rose like a phoenix from the ashes. Denied claims were transformed into rivers of reimbursement, revitalizing the practice's revenue flow and ensuring a brighter future.

The Dance of Documentation

Embark on a journey with a practitioner who unlocked the secrets of meticulous documentation. By harnessing the power of accurate and comprehensive records, this wizard of medical billing banished the specter of claim denials. Denied claims dwindled, and the practice's revenue cycle danced harmoniously, guided by the artistry of thorough documentation.

LESSONS LEARNED AND BEST PRACTICES

The Arcane Art of Persistence

These tales of triumph bear witness to the magic of persistence. Across various challenges and scenarios, a common thread emerges—unyielding dedication to the cause. The road to recovery is paved with tenacity, where even the most stubborn denials can be transformed through unwavering pursuit.

The Elixir of Strategic Partnerships

The case studies reveal the alchemical transformation that occurs when practices join forces with medical billing partners. The power of collaboration and expertise amplifies the potency of recovery efforts, leading to swift and substantial results.

The Sacred Script of Documentation

Within these stories lies the undeniable truth of meticulous documentation. It is the spell that safeguards against claim denials and provides the foundation for successful appeals. Practitioners who master this art wield a powerful weapon against revenue loss.

The Incantation of Communication

Effective communication with payers emerges as a recurring enchantment in these tales. Clear and compelling appeals, coupled with strategic negotiation, hold the power to sway the tides of reimbursement in favor of the practitioner.

The Magic of Data Insight

The journeys of recovery champions are guided by the insights of analytics and reporting. The ability to glean actionable wisdom from recovery data empowers practitioners to make informed decisions, refine strategies, and chart courses to financial prosperity.

The Oath of Ongoing Learning

These stories emphasize the ongoing quest for knowledge and mastery. Just as wizards hone their craft through rigorous study, practitioners in the realm of revenue recovery must remain open to learning, adapting, and embracing new strategies to stay ahead.

As you traverse the landscapes of old accounts receivable recovery, let these tales of success be your guiding stars. Draw inspiration from the triumphs of others and harness the wisdom they offer to illuminate your own path. Through persistence, strategic partnerships, meticulous documentation, effective communication, data insight, and a commitment to ongoing learning, you, too, can script your own success story—one that transforms denied claims into rivers of financial abundance.

CASE STUDIES

Case Study: Unveiling Hidden Revenue Through Strategic Medicaid Engagement

Client Overview:

In the intricate world of medical billing, a healthcare provider found themselves grappling with a persistent challenge – a substantial backlog of unpaid Medicaid claims. Despite meticulous claim submissions, a significant portion remained unreimbursed, leading to revenue loss and financial strain. Operating in Ohio, the provider faced the added complexity of the state's diverse Medicaid coverage options. Desperate for a solution, they turned to the expertise of the Revenue Recovery Wizards.

Challenge: Unpaid Medicaid Claims and Shifting Payer Landscape

The Accounts Receivable (AR) report revealed a concerning pattern of unpaid Medicaid claims that were impacting the provider's financial health. Determined to decipher the root cause, the provider embarked on a journey to uncover the truth behind these lingering unpaid claims. It was soon realized that Ohio's Medicaid landscape offered various payer coverage options, each with distinct member ID numbers and coverage plans. This intricate system presented challenges in aligning claims with the correct payer, leading to revenue leakage.

Discovery: Navigating Complex Payer Changes

Delving deeper, a crucial revelation emerged – effective 3/1/23, one of the Medicaid payers had implemented changes to member ID numbers and coverage details. This coincided with the surge in unpaid claims, creating a direct impact on the provider's revenue stream. The need for immediate intervention to address these changes became paramount.

Solution: Precision and Strategic Payer Engagement

Recognizing the need for a strategic approach, the Revenue Recovery Wizards embarked on a meticulous investigation. Armed with expertise and tenacity, they initiated direct communication with the payer through detailed phone calls. Each conversation aimed to uncover the critical details that had eluded the provider, leading to a deeper understanding of the payer's new system.

Understanding the urgency, the team meticulously researched the previous ID numbers of each patient through the state's Medicaid portal. Simultaneously, they identified and tracked down the new ID numbers brought

91

about by the payer's policy change. This precise data gathering formed the foundation of their strategy.

Implementation: Precision Data Harmonization

Armed with a wealth of meticulously collected data, the Revenue Recovery Wizards executed a dual-pronged strategy. Firstly, they diligently updated the provider's Electronic Health Records (EHR) system with the new ID numbers, ensuring seamless alignment with the payer's modified system. Secondly, outdated ID numbers were systematically retired, paving the way for a smooth transition in future claims submissions.

This harmonization of patient data, member IDs, and coverage details proved transformative. The meticulous effort led to the recovery of hundreds of thousands of dollars for the provider. What initially appeared as an insurmountable challenge was resolved through precision, strategic engagement, and an unwavering commitment to revenue recovery.

Results: Triumph of Expertise and Collaboration

The provider's persistent challenge of unpaid Medicaid claims was not only resolved but transformed into a remarkable success story. The Revenue Recovery Wizards' meticulous approach recouped significant revenue and fortified the provider's future financial stability. This accomplishment highlighted the power of strategic engagement, data precision, and the unwavering dedication to safeguarding revenue streams.

Key Takeaways:

1. Strategic Engagement is Key: The case underscores the importance of strategic communication with payers to unveil hidden challenges and opportunities.

2.   Precision Data Management: The successful resolution hinged on meticulous data collection, alignment, and harmonization.

3.   Expertise Yields Triumph: Expert intervention can transform complex challenges into triumphs, recouping significant revenue and ensuring future financial stability.

Conclusion: Navigating Complexity for Revenue Recovery

The case of unpaid Medicaid claims illustrates the transformative journey from challenge to success, emphasizing the critical role of expertise, precision, and strategic engagement. With the guidance of the Revenue Recovery Wizards, providers can navigate the intricate landscape of medical billing, reclaim lost revenue, and pave the path toward sustained financial vitality.

Case Study: A Strategic Triumph Over Denied Claims with Medical Mutual

Client Overview:

In the intricate landscape of medical billing, even well-established healthcare providers can find themselves grappling with the complexities of claims submission and denial management. This case study sheds light on the journey of a healthcare provider who faced a formidable challenge in addressing denied claims from Medical Mutual. Seeking expert assistance, they turned to the Revenue Recovery Wizards, leading to the successful recovery of $300K in old claims. This case study underscores the power of meticulous investigation, strategic communication, and unwavering persistence.

Challenge: Navigating Complex Denied Claims

The healthcare provider, in partnership with Medical Mutual, encountered a significant roadblock in the form of $300K worth of denied claims. These denials encompassed an array of issues, including sequential order submission non-compliance and type of bill errors. A particularly perplexing challenge emerged – the denial of claims due to apparent missing authorizations. Despite the seemingly straightforward nature of these claims, errors and misalignments had led to significant financial setbacks.

Solution: Meticulous Investigation and Strategic Communication

Recognizing the gravity of the situation, the Revenue Recovery Wizards embarked on a meticulous investigation. They meticulously reviewed each claim, addressing the complexities associated with sequential order submission and type of bill errors. Precision was paramount in ensuring compliance with Medical Mutual's stringent requirements.

For the denied claims rooted in alleged missing authorizations, the Revenue Recovery Wizards delved deeper. Their investigation unveiled a crucial revelation – the authorizations were indeed on file but had not been appropriately linked to the claims. Armed with this insight, the team initiated a detailed call with Medical Mutual's claims supervisor.

Implementation: Bridging Precision and Communication

Through effective communication with the claims supervisor, the Revenue Recovery Wizards sought to rectify the gap between the authorizations and the claims. They presented compelling evidence of the existing authorizations and worked collaboratively to establish the necessary link. In parallel, claims denied due to sequential order submission and type of bill errors were meticulously corrected to align with Medical Mutual's guidelines.

Results: A Resounding Financial Triumph

The meticulous investigation, strategic communication, and precision-driven implementation culminated in an exceptional outcome. The healthcare provider successfully recouped a remarkable $300K in old denied claims that had accumulated over a span of two years. This triumph underscored the significance of timely addressing denied claims and the impact of effective collaboration with payers to rectify errors.

Key Takeaways:

1. Meticulous Investigation: Precision in investigating and understanding the complexities of denied claims is vital for successful recovery.

2. Strategic Communication: Effective communication with payers, like Medical Mutual, is essential to bridge gaps and rectify errors.

3. Unwavering Persistence: Addressing denied claims promptly and persistently can lead to substantial financial recovery and reinforced financial stability.

Conclusion: A Beacon of Expertise and Success

The case study of the provider's journey with Medical Mutual serves as a beacon of expertise and success in the domain of medical billing. The Revenue Recovery Wizards' commitment to precision, communication, and unwavering persistence led to a resounding financial triumph. This case study stands as a testament to the potential of reclaiming denied revenue and strengthening the financial foundation of healthcare providers.

With the Revenue Recovery Wizards as steadfast partners, healthcare providers can navigate the intricate challenges of denied claims, rectify errors with precision, and transform obstacles into opportunities for financial recovery and growth.

Case Study: Navigating Payer Complexities for Substantial Revenue Recovery

Client Overview:

A reputable behavioral health practice was facing a significant challenge with denied claims. Despite submitting claims to the apparent correct payer, they were consistently denied for being directed to the wrong payer.

Challenge: Denied Claims for Incorrect Payer

The practice's billing team diligently submitted claims to the payer they believed was responsible for medical services. However, these claims were met with denials for "incorrect payer." This puzzling trend was causing not only financial strain but also frustration among the practice's team.

Discovery: Carve-Out Payer Arrangement

In-depth research by the revenue recovery experts revealed a subtle but crucial detail: the patient's medical plan featured a 'carve-out' provision for behavioral health services. This meant that behavioral health claims were directed to a separate payer, unbeknownst to the practice's billing team.

Solution: A Pivotal Clarification Call

Understanding the importance of precise payer information, the Revenue Recovery Wizards initiated a call to the medical payer. Their goal was to clarify the correct payer responsible for processing behavioral health claims. After an insightful conversation with the payer's representative, the accurate payer details were finally obtained.

Results: Over $100,000 in Revenue Recovery

With the correct payer information in hand, the practice's billing team resubmitted the denied claims to the designated payer for behavioral health services. The claims were promptly processed and accepted, leading to a remarkable recovery of over one hundred thousand dollars in revenue that would have otherwise been lost.

Key Takeaways:

1. Precision in Payer Identification: The case underscored the significance of accurately identifying the correct payer, especially in situations involving specialized carve-out arrangements.

2. Proactive Communication: Initiating communication with payers, even in complex cases, can yield essential insights that lead to successful revenue recovery.

3. Expertise Matters: Utilizing the expertise of revenue recovery professionals can unravel complex payer intricacies and maximize financial

gains for healthcare practices.

Conclusion:

This case exemplifies how even the smallest nuances in payer arrangements can have a substantial impact on claims processing and revenue recovery. Through proactive investigation, clear communication, and expert insights, the behavioral health practice not only resolved their denied claims but also unlocked a significant stream of revenue, reinforcing the value of industry expertise and dedication to financial success.

Case Study: Maximizing Revenue Recovery through Expert Toxicology Billing

Client Overview:

A prominent healthcare facility faced a formidable challenge as its in-house billing team grappled with the overwhelming task of processing inpatient and outpatient facility claims. The complexity of coding and applying modifiers to toxicology claims further compounded the team's struggle. Seeking professional guidance, they turned to the Revenue Recovery Wizards for assistance.

Challenge: Overwhelmed Billing Team and Complex Toxicology Billing

The in-house billing team found themselves drowning in a sea of inpatient and outpatient facility claims, unable to cope with the sheer volume. Adding to their predicament were the toxicology claims, which posed intricate coding and modifier challenges. The billing team's lack of expertise in this area left these claims untouched, contributing to substantial revenue loss.

Discovery: Unveiling Hidden Revenue Potential

Recognizing the untapped potential for revenue recovery, the healthcare facility enlisted the expertise of the Revenue Recovery Wizards. With their specialized knowledge of toxicology billing, the experts understood the intricate coding nuances and the critical role of appropriate modifiers. Upon delving into the situation, they uncovered a pivotal revelation – the in-house billing team was solely focusing on high-dollar claims, oblivious to the treasure trove of low-dollar toxicology claims.

Solution: Unlocking the Power of Expert Toxicology Billing

The Revenue Recovery Wizards embarked on a transformative journey to address the pressing challenges. Armed with their proficiency in toxicology coding and modifiers, they meticulously navigated through each claim. They embarked on an initiative to code and apply the necessary modifiers to toxicology claims, ensuring their accurate submission.

Results: $1.5 Million in Recouped Revenue and Unveiling Hidden Potential

Leveraging their expertise, the Revenue Recovery Wizards embarked on a comprehensive endeavor to tackle the full spectrum of claims, toxicology included, spanning back 12 months. This strategic move led to a staggering $1.5 million in recovered revenue. What initially appeared as low-dollar claims amassed into a substantial financial gain, underscoring the latent potential within overlooked claims.

Key Takeaways:

1.   Expertise Unlocks Revenue: The   case

emphasizes the transformative impact of expertise in navigating intricate coding and modifier requirements, particularly in areas like toxicology.

2.   Inclusivity Matters: Addressing all claims, regardless of their individual value, can result in significant revenue recovery, even from seemingly insignificant claims.

3.   Strategic Collaboration: Partnering with revenue recovery experts empowers healthcare facilities to harness hidden revenue potential and optimize claims processing.

Conclusion:

This case exemplifies the profound influence of expert intervention in grappling with complex claims processing and revenue recovery challenges. By harnessing the expertise of the Revenue Recovery Wizards, the healthcare facility not only reclaimed substantial toxicology revenue but also unveiled the power of inclusive claims management. The narrative underscores the pivotal role of expertise and strategic collaboration in uncovering untapped financial opportunities.

Case Study: Resolving Denied Claims Through Expert Negotiation with Tribal Council

Client Overview:

Navigating the intricate realm of medical billing, a healthcare provider encountered a persistent challenge of denied claims due to medical necessity review requirements. Despite diligent efforts, these denials resulted in continued delays and revenue loss. Seeking resolution, the provider turned to the expertise of the Revenue Recovery Wizards.

Challenge: Denials and Delays Due to Medical Necessity Review

The provider faced recurring denials for claims requiring medical necessity review. This challenge not only caused revenue leakage but also contributed to ongoing delays in processing claims. The team was determined to overcome this hurdle and recoup the revenue lost due to denials.

Discovery: Payer Referral to Tribal Council

In the pursuit of a solution, the Revenue Recovery Wizards initiated a call to the payer responsible for the denied claims. During this communication, the payer directed the team's attention to a unique situation – the claims were being referred to a tribal council for further review. This referral added an additional layer of complexity to the case.

Solution: Strategic Engagement with Tribal Council

Armed with this newfound knowledge, the Revenue Recovery Wizards embarked on a detailed phone call with a claims supervisor at the tribal council. The objective was to understand the reasons behind the denials and explore potential avenues for resolution. The conversation revealed that the tribal council acknowledged the need for medical care but faced financial constraints preventing them from funding the claims at the billed amount.

Implementation: Expert Negotiation for Mutual Agreement

Recognizing the importance of resolving this impasse, the

revenue recovery experts initiated a negotiation. They worked collaboratively with the tribal council to find a middle ground that would benefit both parties. The negotiation aimed to determine an acceptable payment amount that would allow the tribal council to provide care while addressing the provider's revenue loss.

Results: A Successful Resolution and Financial Recovery

The negotiation bore fruit as a mutually agreeable fee was settled upon. Instead of facing a complete denial, the provider achieved a significant victory. The tribal council agreed to pay $42,000, a substantial recovery compared to the original billed amount of $84,000. This outcome showcased the transformative impact of strategic negotiation and expert engagement.

Key Takeaways:

1. Expert Negotiation: The case emphasizes the power of expert negotiation in navigating complex denials and finding mutually beneficial solutions.

2. Collaborative Approach: Collaboration between providers and payers, even in unique situations like tribal council review, can lead to successful resolutions.

3. Persistence Pays Off: The Revenue Recovery Wizards' persistence in engaging with payers and finding common ground resulted in substantial financial recovery.

Conclusion: Triumph Through Expert Engagement

This case exemplifies the pivotal role of expert

intervention and negotiation in overcoming denied claims and recovering lost revenue. By leveraging their expertise, the Revenue Recovery Wizards not only resolved the challenge but also transformed it into a significant financial victory. This narrative underscores the value of collaboration, persistence, and strategic negotiation in the realm of medical billing, ultimately reinforcing the financial stability of healthcare providers.

Case Study: Unraveling Complex Bundling Issues to Unlock Hidden Revenue

Client Overview:

In the intricate landscape of medical billing, a healthcare provider faced a perplexing challenge stemming from bundled codes and denied claims. Specifically, they encountered complications with BCBS OH's coding regulations, where toxicology code G0481 was bundled with 80307, leading to denials. Seeking resolution, the provider turned to the Revenue Recovery Wizards for expertise and guidance.

Challenge: Complex Coding and Bundling Denials

The provider grappled with the complex coding dynamics involving toxicology code G0481 and code 80307, as stipulated by BCBS OH. Their efforts to bill G0481 separately were met with denials, causing revenue leakage. The situation was further exacerbated by the payer's decision to stop reimbursing for G0481 claims altogether. The provider lacked the necessary time and resources to untangle this intricate web of bundled codes and denied claims.

Discovery: Uncovering Hidden Revenue Potential

Upon delving into the provider's Accounts Receivable (AR), the Revenue Recovery Wizards unearthed a substantial amount tied to G0481 claims. Recognizing the potential for revenue recovery, they embarked on a detailed research endeavor to decipher the payer's medical policy that was contributing to the denials.

Solution: Navigating Bundling Dynamics and Code Alternatives

Through meticulous research and data analysis, the revenue recovery experts uncovered the key to resolving the challenge. They identified that when G0481 was billed on the same date as 80307, the payer bundled the codes together, resulting in denials for G0481. To navigate this issue, the solution was to bill a less comprehensive code, G0480, which allowed for separate billing alongside 80307. Despite G0480's lower reimbursement rate of $27, the sheer volume of claims made it a promising alternative.

Implementation: Optimizing Claims Processing for Revenue Recovery

Armed with this insight, the Revenue Recovery Wizards collaborated closely with the provider's billing team to implement the solution. They strategically transitioned from billing G0481 to G0480, ensuring that it was billed alongside 80307 to maximize revenue potential.

Results: Unleashing Substantial Revenue Recovery

The strategic shift from G0481 to G0480, coupled with accurate billing alongside 80307, bore remarkable results. Despite the lower reimbursement rate of $27, the significant volume of claims accumulated to a substantial revenue recovery of over $50,000. This outcome showcased the transformative impact of precise coding strategy and expert intervention.

Key Takeaways:

1. Strategic Code Transition: The case underscores the importance of strategically transitioning to alternative codes to overcome bundling denials and maximize revenue potential.

2. Expert Research: In-depth research into payer policies and coding dynamics is crucial for uncovering hidden revenue opportunities.

3. Sheer Volume Matters: Even when dealing with lower reimbursement rates, the cumulative effect of addressing a large number of claims can lead to substantial revenue recovery.

Conclusion: Triumph Through Expert Intervention

This case exemplifies the profound influence of expert intervention in overcoming complex coding challenges and unlocking hidden revenue. By leveraging their expertise, the Revenue Recovery Wizards not only resolved the issue but also transformed it into a significant financial victory. This narrative underscores the value of meticulous research, strategic coding, and the collaborative effort between healthcare providers and revenue recovery experts in navigating the intricacies of medical billing.

ACTION ITEMS

1. Conduct a thorough analysis of unpaid claims to identify patterns and trends.

2. Implement a process to regularly review Accounts Receivable (AR) reports for unpaid claims.

3. Develop a strategy to address denied claims promptly and strategically.

4. Establish direct communication channels with payers to clarify claim denials and changes in policies.

5. Create a team specializing in investigating denied claims and payer intricacies.

6. Ensure meticulous documentation of payer policy changes and their effective dates.

7. Implement a process to cross-reference patient ID numbers with payer changes to prevent misalignments.

8. Regularly update Electronic Health Records (EHR) with new payer information to ensure accurate claims submission.

9. Retire outdated patient ID numbers from the system to prevent future misalignments.

10. Develop a system for tracking and addressing changes in payer coverage options.

11. Train billing teams on specific payer policies, including carve-out arrangements.

12. Establish a direct line of communication with payer representatives for clarifications.

13. Utilize data analysis to identify potential revenue leakage due to payer complexities.

14. Collaborate with payer representatives to ensure authorizations are accurately linked to claims.

15. Establish a systematic approach for tracking and resolving sequential order submissions and type of bill errors.

16. Leverage expert assistance to address toxicology billing challenges, including coding and modifiers.

17. Implement a process for accurately coding and applying modifiers to both high-dollar and low-dollar claims.

18. Regularly review and update the billing team's knowledge of coding and billing intricacies.

19. Create a protocol for reviewing claims that are left unprocessed due to coding complexities.

20. Consider partnering with Revenue Recovery Wizards to optimize claims processing and revenue recovery efforts.

YOUR ROADMAP TO FINANCIAL HEALTH

CREATING A SUSTAINABLE REVENUE RECOVERY PROCESS

In the enchanted realm of medical billing, where the arcane arts of revenue recovery converge with the dance of unpaid claims, crafting a roadmap to financial health becomes a sacred quest. With each step, practitioners journey toward a realm where the currency of persistence, wisdom, and transformation reigns supreme. Within this chapter, we unveil the blueprint for your own odyssey toward a sustainable revenue recovery process, where the heartbeats of ongoing improvement resonate like an ancient incantation.

CULTIVATING A CULTURE OF ONGOING IMPROVEMENT

Like ancient alchemists who tirelessly sought the philosopher's stone, your journey to financial health begins with a pledge to constant growth. Within this chapter of your saga, the importance of fostering a culture of ongoing improvement takes center stage—a culture where every team member becomes an apprentice to the art of transformation.

The Alchemical Mindset

Within the crucible of your practice, the seeds of ongoing improvement are sown by embracing an alchemical mindset. Just as base metals can be transformed into gold, so too can unresolved accounts be transmuted into reclaimed revenue. Encourage your team to view each challenge as an opportunity for refinement, each setback as a catalyst for innovation.

The Forge of Collaborative Mastery

Forge a fellowship of collaboration, where each member of your practice becomes a craftsman in the workshop of recovery. Foster an environment where ideas flow freely, where insights are shared openly, and where the collective genius of your team is harnessed to overcome obstacles and seize opportunities.

The Cauldron of Data Wisdom

Within the cauldron of data lies the elixir of foresight. Teach your team to distill wisdom from the pools of information you gather, transforming raw data into strategic insight. Let them become the seers who predict trends, unveiling patterns that guide your journey toward financial prosperity.

The Grimoire of Education

Empower your practitioners with the grimoire of knowledge. Encourage them to become lifelong learners, always seeking to deepen their understanding of the ever-evolving landscape of medical billing. Provide opportunities for training, workshops, and continuous education, enabling them to wield a wider array of spells in the art of recovery.

The Enchanted Ritual of Feedback

Infuse the practice with the magic of feedback. Regularly convene gatherings where experiences are shared, lessons are learned, and insights are celebrated. By engaging in this ritual, your team conjures a space where collective wisdom flourishes and individual growth is nurtured.

The Quest for Innovation

Kindled by the spirit of discovery, your practitioners embark on a quest for innovative solutions. Encourage them to explore new strategies, experiment with novel approaches, and push the boundaries of convention. Just as the alchemists of old sought hidden truths, your team will uncover fresh paths to revenue recovery.

As you etch the runes of ongoing improvement into the tapestry of your practice, remember that the art of transformation is a journey, not a destination. Like the sages of old, who tirelessly pursued the elusive elixir of life, your dedication to perpetual growth holds the key to unlocking the gates of financial health. Through each cycle of improvement, each breakthrough, and each triumph, you weave a legacy of prosperity that endures through the ages—a legacy that transforms your practice into a haven of thriving abundance.

ACTION ITEMS

1. **Assess Current Recovery Process:** Evaluate your current old AR recovery process and identify areas that need improvement. Gather data on recovery success rates, timeframes, and any recurring challenges.

2. **Set Clear Recovery Goals:** Define specific, measurable, achievable, relevant, and time-bound (SMART) goals for your old AR recovery efforts. Consider factors such as recovery rates, reduction in denials, and improved revenue flow.

3. **Prioritize and Segment Accounts:** Categorize old AR accounts based on factors like age, payer type, and denial reasons. Prioritize accounts with the highest potential for recovery and design targeted strategies for each segment.

4. **Develop a Comprehensive Strategy:** Create a structured recovery plan that outlines the steps to be taken for each account segment. Incorporate lessons learned from case studies and best practices from previous chapters.

5. **Allocate Resources and Responsibilities:** Assign specific roles and responsibilities to team members involved in the recovery process. Allocate necessary resources, including time, technology, and training, to ensure successful execution.

6. **Implement Process Improvements:** Introduce process improvements based on best practices to enhance the efficiency of your old AR recovery efforts. Streamline workflows, reduce bottlenecks, and incorporate automation where applicable.

7. **Regular Monitoring and Analysis:** Establish a

system for continuous monitoring of recovery progress. Analyze key performance indicators (KPIs) to measure the effectiveness of your strategies.

8. **Adjust Strategies as Needed:** Remain flexible and willing to adjust strategies based on real-time data and feedback. If certain approaches aren't yielding the expected results, adapt and pivot as necessary.

9. **Ongoing Training and Education:** Provide ongoing training and education to your team members to keep them updated on industry changes and best practices. Encourage continuous learning to maintain a high level of expertise.

10. **Celebrate Milestones and Achievements:** Recognize and celebrate successes as you achieve your recovery goals. Use these moments to boost morale and reinforce the positive impact of your efforts.

11. **Regularly Review and Update the Roadmap:** Set regular intervals for reviewing and updating your recovery roadmap to ensure its relevance. Incorporate new insights and adjust strategies based on evolving challenges and opportunities.

12. **Foster a Culture of Improvement:** Promote a culture of continuous improvement within your team. Encourage open communication, idea sharing, and collaboration to optimize recovery processes.

By following these action items, you'll be able to create a roadmap that guides your practice toward financial health through effective old AR recovery. This chapter will empower you with a structured approach to consistently enhance your recovery efforts, achieve your goals, and maintain a thriving revenue cycle.

EPILOGUE: EMBRACING YOUR LEGACY OF FINANCIAL VITALITY

As we draw the final curtain on this mystical journey through the realms of old accounts receivable recovery, you, dear practitioner, stand at the crossroads of transformation. The chapters preceding this epilogue have unfurled a tapestry of wisdom, guiding you through the arcane arts of revenue reclamation, the dance of denied claims, and the incantations of recovery success. Yet, this is not the end, but the beginning—an initiation into a legacy of financial vitality that will echo through time.

In the realm of medical billing, the quest for unrecovered revenue is perpetual, an ever-turning wheel of opportunity that allows you to mend the frayed threads of your practice's financial health. You have been bestowed with the knowledge to decipher the ancient codes of claims, to unravel the intricacies of insurance, and to summon forth the magic of effective communication. With each learned lesson, you have transformed into a true maestro of the recovery symphony, guiding your practice toward the crescendo of prosperity.

As you tread the path ahead, remember that your journey does not end here. The Ultimate Guide to Old Accounts Receivable Recovery is not a mere tome to gather dust on a shelf—it is your spellbook, a key to unlock the doors of abundance. Let its pages be your compass, guiding you through the labyrinth of denials and leading you toward the hidden treasures of reclaimed revenue.

Embrace the lessons learned from the success stories and case studies, letting them fuel your determination to surmount every obstacle. Harness the power of ongoing improvement, allowing it to infuse your practice with the spirit of transformation. Stand firm in the face of denials, armed with the knowledge that each challenge is a steppingstone toward greater financial health.

As the final chapter of this guide draws to a close, you are not bidding farewell to an adventure, but embarking on a new phase of your saga—one where your practice flourishes, your revenue soars, and your legacy of financial vitality becomes an enduring testament to your dedication and wisdom.

Remember, practitioner, that the arcane arts of old accounts receivable recovery are yours to wield. With each incantation of insight, each infusion of wisdom, and each spark of innovation, you shape your own destiny—a destiny of prosperity, growth, and success.

The magic is yours to command. Go forth and weave your legacy.

In gratitude and triumph,

The Revenue Recovery Wizards

UNLEASH THE MAGIC OF REVENUE RECOVERY

Unleash the Magic of Revenue Recovery with a FREE 40-minute Revenue Recovery Consultation!

Are you ready to witness the enchanting transformation of your practice's financial realm?

Prepare to be spellbound by a personalized 40-minute exploration of your accounts receivable, guided by our Revenue Recovery Wizards – and the most bewitching part?

It's absolutely FREE!

We possess such mystical confidence in our ability to conjure revenue that we're offering this risk-free opportunity to unveil the hidden treasures within your dormant claims.

During Your FREE Consultation, You'll Experience

1. **Sorcery of Hidden Revenue Streams:** Watch in awe as we reveal the arcane sources of revenue tucked away in your accounts receivable, ready to

emerge as a splendid financial boon.

2. **Wizardry Tailored to You:** Behold our enchanting spells, custom-crafted to breathe life into your old accounts, transforming lingering claims into shimmering coins of realized revenue.

3. **Magic Pact of Performance:** Experience the tranquil assurance of our "no recovery, no fee" pledge – witness the mystical bond where payment is conjured only when we conjure back funds for you.

4. **Efficiency Elixirs:** Immerse yourself in the elixirs of wisdom, as we unveil mystical insights to streamline your accounts receivable, banishing delays and ushering in a river of flowing gold.

5. **Enchanted Compliance:** Gaze upon our mastery of ethical financial enchantments, ensuring your practice dances in harmony with industry-ethereal forces.

6. **Personalized Incantations:** Depart with a personalized incantation – a mystical roadmap tailored to your practice, guiding you on a journey to financial ascension and prosperity.

Release the shackles of uncollected revenue and embark on a journey of arcane financial revelation. Secure your spot for the FREE 40-minute consultation, and together, we shall conjure greater revenue, restore the balance of cash flow, and etch your practice's name among the stars of financial triumph.

The power of your potential, woven with our wizardry – let the magic unfold!

While there is still time, book a free consultation at www.RevenueRecoveryWizards.com.

If you prefer, scan the QR code to book a call.

Of course, the choice is yours.

THE REVENUE RECOVERY WIZARDS

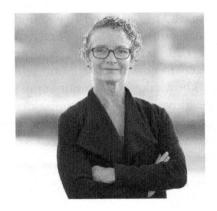

REBECCA HOLLINGER

Rebecca Hollinger brings a wealth of expertise in Revenue Cycle Management (RCM) and medical billing, gained through a dynamic career spanning over two decades. Her extensive experience and dedication to the healthcare industry make her a true asset in the field.

Rebecca's role as Assistant Director of Revenue Cycle Management showcases her specialization in claim denial and rejection management. She demonstrates a keen understanding of both In- and Out-of-Network provider reimbursement across various payer types, including commercial, Medicaid, Medicare, and behavioral health carve-outs. Rebecca's meticulous approach has led to the timely billing of over 100,000 claims, generating substantial revenue from toxicology and COVID-19 testing claims under key accounts.

Her expertise extends to training and mentoring staff on various RCM practices, creating a culture of excellence and expertise within her team. She is a driving force behind billing strategies that align with payer guidelines, ensuring maximum revenue recovery and operational efficiency.

Rebecca's role as an RCM Manager at LTC Billing Solutions showcased her comprehensive understanding of billing guidelines and rates for Medicare A and B, Medicaid, and commercial payers. She trained facility personnel to excel in administrative and billing functions, imparting her knowledge of benefit limits, CPT codes, timely filing deadlines, and COB requirements. Rebecca's meticulous attention to detail translated into accurate AR reviews, Excel reports, and effective AR collections, ensuring proper payment of claims.

With her comprehensive expertise in RCM, medical billing, and business management, Rebecca Hollinger is a beacon of knowledge and professionalism. Her commitment to accuracy, strategic thinking, and team development has positively impacted countless medical practices, resulting in enhanced revenue recovery and operational excellence.

For further insights or to explore how Rebecca's expertise can benefit your medical practice, reach out to her at rebecca@rebeccahollinger.com or visit our website at www.RevenueRecoveryWizards.com.

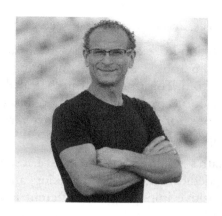

DON KERMATH

Don Kermath is a dynamic professional with a wealth of experience across diverse fields, showcasing a unique blend of entrepreneurship, leadership, technical expertise, and passion for business systems. With a solid foundation in architecture and management, Don has made remarkable contributions to various industries throughout his career.

Don's journey as an entrepreneur and visionary leader encompasses roles in various organizations spanning multiple domains. Don has become an employee turnover reduction and business systems expert.

Don Kermath has authored several impactful publications, ranging from books to reports, covering subjects like employee management, small business strategies, indoor air quality, historic preservation, and more. These publications reflect his commitment to sharing knowledge and insights across diverse fields.

Don Kermath's commitment to continuous learning is evident through his Master of Architecture degree and participation in various managerial and technical workshops, seminars, and training programs. He has also been actively involved in professional organizations, leadership roles, and community service.

Don's dedication to excellence has been acknowledged through numerous awards, including leadership recognition from Toastmasters International, certificates of appreciation from various organizations, and commendations for his contributions to various projects and initiatives.

Don Kermath's multifaceted career is a testament to his unwavering dedication, strategic thinking, and passion for making a positive impact across different industries. His journey highlights his role as a visionary entrepreneur, educator, author, and advocate for small and medium-sized businesses.

For further insights or to explore how Don's expertise can benefit your medical practice, reach out to him at don@donkermath.com or visit our website at www.RevenueRecoveryWizards.com.

Made in the USA
Middletown, DE
17 March 2024

51048215R00070